D0153971

Leadership for Nursing and Allied Health Care Professions

Leadership for Nursing and Allied Health Care Professions

Editor: Veronica Bishop

 Open University Press

BP45

Open University Press
McGraw-Hill Education
McGraw-Hill House
Shoppenhangers Road
Maidenhead
Berkshire
England
SL6 2QL

email: enquiries@openup.co.uk
world wide web: www.openup.co.uk

and Two Penn Plaza, New York, NY 10121—2289, USA

First published 2009

A catalogue record of this book is available from the British Library

ISBN-13: 9780335225330 (pb) 978033522532-3 (hb)
ISBN-10: 033522533-0 (pb) 033522532-2 (hb)

Typeset by Kerrypress, Luton, Bedfordshire
Printed and bound in the UK by Bell and Bain Ltd.

Mixed Sources
Product group from well-managed
forests and other controlled sources
www.fsc.org Cert no. TT-COC-002769
© 1996 Forest Stewardship Council
FSC

The **McGraw·Hill** Companies

11/23/09

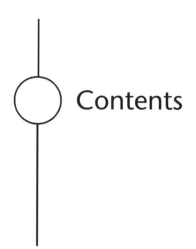

Contents

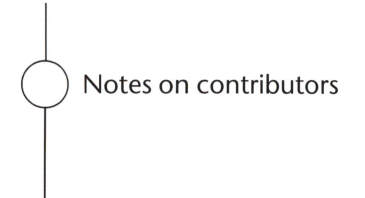

Notes on contributors

Sue Antrobus, MPhil, BSc, PGDipEd, RGN, has over 20 years' experience working with, or connected to, the National Health Service (NHS), the independent sector, academia and a major professional union. In her NHS work she has held roles in the Department of Health and with health authorities and has worked directly with patients in clinical practice. Sue currently holds a non-executive appointment at a primary care trust in the north west of England, where she has the non-executive lead for commissioning, patient safety and clinical quality. Her particular interest throughout her career has been to enable health and social care staff to contribute effectively at a strategic and policy level through leadership development. She has a particular interest in commissioning and has worked at a national policy level to develop the nursing contribution to the commissioning agenda. As a successful change agent, Sue has a renowned track record of working with a range of partners to agree priorities and translate those into programmes that bring about service improvement and change across the UK and internationally.

Veronica Bishop, PhD, MPhil, RGN, FRSA, is Visiting Professor of Nursing at City University, London, editor-in-chief of the *Journal of Research in Nursing* (Sage) and a Fellow of the Royal Society of Arts. She is an adviser to the *Hong Kong Nursing Journal*, a member of the scientific committee for the Royal College of Nursing (RCN) Research Society, and until recently an executive member of the Florence Nightingale Foundation and a member of its academic panel. Veronica came late into nursing after a varied career. Having gained her RGN and specialized in cardio-thoracic and intensive care nursing, she joined the Anaesthetic Research Department at the Royal College of Surgeons (England) and obtained an MPhil (CNAA), followed by a PhD through the Faculty of Medicine, London University. Both degrees sought to bridge the gap between clinical research and nursing. She then joined the Civil Service as a nursing officer where she had responsibility for a large body of nursing and midwifery research and workforce studies for the entire NHS. She also had the national lead across the UK for clinical supervision, and commissioned the first national multi-site study in nursing. Veronica has worked as a consultant for the WHO in Denmark, India and Romania, is widely published and has presented keynote speeches at numerous nursing conferences.

Philip Esterhuizen, PhD, MScN, BA, is a nursing lecturer in research and elective English-language modules on intercultural sensitivity in the Netherlands. He is involved in Master's and Bachelor curriculum development, and supervises students at Doctoral and Master's levels. Between 2002 and 2008 he worked in academic settings in England and ran action research in various settings, was involved in developing or sustaining clinical supervision and was curriculum development consultant and an external panel member validating undergraduate, postgraduate and Master's programmes, at two universities in Ireland. Philip reviews manuscripts for numerous international journals. His PhD research explored the socialization and professional development of undergraduate nursing students in the Netherlands.

Dawn Freshwater, PhD, BA, RNT, RN, FRCN, is Professor and Dean of the School of Health care at the University of Leeds, a Fellow of the Royal College of Nursing and editor of the *Journal of Psychiatric Mental Health Nursing*. She is an active member of Sigma Theta Tau receiving the Distinguished Researcher Award in 2000, and is an executive member of the Florence Nightingale Foundation, where she sits on the research scholarship panel. Since the early 1990s she has maintained an interest in the application and evaluation of transformational research, critical reflexivity, pragmatism, reflective practice and clinical supervision, and in particular its relation to evidence-based practice and the therapeutic alliance. She is external reviewer for the Forensic Mental Health Fellowships and sits on a number of international grant review panels. Dawn is a prolific writer and passionate about developing leadership capacity through high quality research and education. In this context she has a particular interest in transformational leadership, reflective practice and strategic planning. She has undertaken significant strategic change in her current role and was nominated as a woman of achievement in 2008.

Tyrone Goh, DSc, MBA, FCR, FIR (Aust.), HDCR, TDCR, is a radiographer who moved into mainstream health care management. He is the current executive director of three business units in Singapore, at the National Health care Group (NHG), which operates the largest primary care diagnostic service in the country and performs health care consultancy to regional countries. Tyrone was made an honorary Doctor of Science at South Bank University, London, where he is a Visiting Fellow. Tyrone is recognized at the highest level by many governments as well as his own, and a champion of the radiography profession and the service worldwide. He is past president of the International Society of Radiographers and sits on several local boards in academia and hospitals. Some of Tyrone's achievements include setting up a radiotherapy centre at Singapore's National University Hospital and initiating the first island-wide tele-radiology service in Singapore. He has been given several local and international awards, and awarded the commendation medal by the President of Singapore, and the National Health care Group distinguished staff achievement award, the highest accolade given to non-clinical staff.

Iain Graham, PhD, MSc, MEd, BSc, RGN, RMN, is Professor of Nursing and Head of School, Health and Human Sciences Faculty of Arts and Sciences, Southern Cross University, NSW, Australia. He is a registered nurse in both the UK and New South Wales, and qualified as a mental health nurse in the UK. Iain has a background in advanced clinical practice, health service management and education and has held various academic and service positions in the UK. He is an Adjunct Professor in Nursing to Vanderbilt University, Nashville, Tennessee, University of Northumbria, UK, and University of Technology, Sydney, and holds fellowships with the European Academy of Nurse Scientists and the Royal Society of Health. During 2005–2007, Iain was President of the Consortium of Higher Education, Health and Rehabilitation Educators, a European-based organization promoting inter-professional education with health care. He teaches in the areas of leadership, nursing theory and health policy, and supervises students at doctoral and master's levels.

Mary Lovegrove, MSc, TDCR, HDCR, DMU, DCR(R), MSSR, is a diagnostic radiographer by profession, Professor of Education and Development for Allied Health Professions, and very involved in the world of AHP. She is Head of Department of Allied Health Sciences at London South Bank University (LSBU) and a Director of Centre for Research in AHP at LSBU. Mary balances her time between local, national and international activities. She is an adviser to the UK Department of Health on Allied Health Development issues and to the Health Authority of Hong Kong; she is a member of London Higher and of the NHS London Education and Workforce review advisory committee. She previously served as the vice-president for the International Society of Radiographers and Radiological Technologists (Europe and Africa) and is an honorary member of the Singapore Society of Radiographers. Mary is an Allied Health Executive Member for the UK Council of Deans for Nursing and Health Professions and is a member of the NHS London AHP Network Steering Committee.

Annie Macleod, RCN, RM, MPhil, BSc, is currently a senior manager with Hull Teaching Primary Care Trust. She is a nurse and midwife and has over 20 years' experience in the NHS in service redesign, project management, organizational development and evaluation research. She has worked with the RCN to complete a Department of Health sponsored national evaluation of the clinical leadership programme. Since 2003, Annie has evaluated the political leadership programme, which has been delivered to a variety of national and international participants.

Abigail Masterson, MPA, MN, BSc, PGCEA, RN, FRSA, is Assistant Director Clinical Quality at the Health Foundation and also director of her own consultancy company. Abigail's work ranges from national level projects involving many powerful stakeholder groups to small service and/or organizational development work in individual health and voluntary sector organizations. She has worked with frontline clinical staff as well as senior managers and policy staff from the full range of professions and disciplines in health and social care.

Mike Saks, PhD, MA, BA, studied at the University of Lancaster, the University of Kent and the London School of Economics, where he obtained a BA, MA and PhD in sociology respectively. After taking up a lecturer post at De Montfort University, he successively became Head of Department, Head of School and Dean of the Faculty of Health and Community Studies. He is currently Professor and Senior Pro Vice Chancellor at the University of Lincoln. Mike has published widely on professionalization, health care and complementary and alternative medicine, and given many keynote presentations at national and international conferences. He has served on a wide range of NHS committees at local, regional and national level and acted as a consultant to professional bodies in health care and the UK Department of Health. Mike has been involved in a number of international research collaborations and is currently President of the International Sociological Association Research Committee on Professional Groups.

David Stanley, D.Nurs, MSc, BN, RGN, RM, began his career in nursing when it was deemed vocational and was steeped in tradition. Since then he has seen the transition of nursing into a proud and evidence-based profession. He trained as a registered nurse and midwife in South Australia and worked through his formative career in a number of hospitals and clinical environments there. In 1993 he completed a Bachelor of Nursing at Flinders University, Adelaide (for which he was awarded the university medal). After a number of years as a volunteer midwife in Africa, he moved to the UK to work as the co-ordinator of children's services in York, and as a nurse practitioner. In pursuit of clinical excellence he completed a master's in health science at Birmingham University. After a short return to Australia where he was director of nursing for remote health services in Alice Springs,

David returned to the UK to complete his Nursing Doctorate. This focused on his research on clinical leadership. He is currently living in Perth, Western Australia.

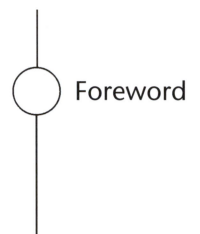

Foreword

I am delighted to write a foreword to this most timely publication.

Leadership is very much at the centre of debates about the delivery of health care. At the time of writing this foreword there are significant policy proposals emerging that will influence health care leadership in England. These proposals have strong resonances in other parts of the UK and the rest of the world.

The 'Next Stage Review' (Department of Health 2008) report is a product of Lord Darzi's recent extensive examination of health care provision for England. It has provided renewed focus on clinician – led services and, more importantly for this book and its readers, it suggests a central and critical role for leaders drawn from the nursing and allied health professions.

There have been recent suggestions that some of the health care professions and nursing in particular has 'lost its way'. This narrow attempt to lay blame for inadequate service provision ignores a broader view held by others who suggest that the whole of the health care system has lost its way, blinded by the urgent pursuit of targets, 'must do' efficiency measures and insensitive executive authority.

Not that the health professions are blameless. They have lacked strong leaders that could have urged and led a necessary counter-culture and kept patients and families at the very centre of health care provision. Such a counter force is notably scarce and it is affected by a predominance of leadership styles that have sometimes stalled the development of modern clinical services. The emphasis has largely been upon more traditional models of management when innovative services require leadership that will embrace those traditions, but is further enriched by clinical experience. This may not be well articulated as yet, but we might do worse than listen to the advice of Hills (2004) who suggests that implicit knowledge – that which grows from personal experience, and explicit knowledge – that which grows from the more formal acquisition of knowledge, has equal value. He argues that 'the value of explicit knowledge lies not in its ownership but in its application. If explicit knowledge is the basis of the human intellect then the implicit kind is the basis of human intelligence.' It follows then that the implicit knowledge of the nurse and allied health professional must be consciously used, in tandem with, and not overwhelmed by, clever science and management theories. Through this, nurses and allied health professionals will have value as leaders who will truly add benefit the delivery of services.

Thankfully, new (or renewed) vocabulary is gaining ascendancy. Patient centredness, clinical leadership, compassion and patient safety are the revitalized cornerstones of health care provision. The underpinning values of health care systems are also being re-stated. In the United Kingdom these will be expressed as a set of core values for the United Kingdom National Health Service. These renewed values will bear down on the provision of health care but will not be realized properly unless driven by influential leadership from nurses and allied health professionals. The Kings College National Nursing Research Unit has produced a thoughtful document (Maben and Griffiths 2008) which seeks to stimulate further debate and suggests that 'our professionalism needs to be underpinned by a reinvigorated sense of service'.

Underpining the new mood there are influential organizations who seek to play their part. In the UK a proposed National Leadership Council led by the NHS Chief Executive and a Faculty for Innovation and Improvement (under the auspices of the NHS Institute for Innovation and Improvement) will soon emerge. The Institute for Health Improvement in the USA has also played a continuous role in leadership development across the world.

There are, of course, strong impressive leaders already drawn from nursing and health professions but they are in short supply and the next generation of these 'best of the best' must be purposefully found and nurtured, not serendipitously uncovered. There have been noble attempts to make a difference through professional organizations such as the UK Royal College of Nursing. One of the problems besetting such imaginative leadership programmes is when their inspired and equipped aspirant leaders have returned to work they have been discouraged from leading organizational changes. The Chief Executives of health care organizations bear a responsibility to be sure that that this waste of talent and investment does not continue.

The climate is ripe for change and clearly, this book could not be timelier. The editor and her contributing authors are to be congratulated for its production.

For those nurses and allied health professionals seeking to take their place as leaders it will provide both a stimulus and a creditable source of reference.

The selection of subject areas is commendable, interesting case studies make strong illustrations and arguments about the nature of leadership and its importance are made with authority. The book is most welcome and provides an intelligent platform, helpfully and cleverly informing the clamour for new leaders, particularly for those drawn from clinicians and practitioners.

I applaud this excellent publication, and see its contribution as long overdue.

References

Department of Health (2008). A high quality workforce: NHS Next Stage Review. London: DoH.

Hills, G. (2004) In from the cold – the rise of vocational education. *Journal of the Royal Society of Arts,* November.

Maben, J. and Griffiths, P. (2008) *Nurses in Society: starting the debate.* National Nursing Research Unit. London: Kings College.

Tony Butterworth CBE
Emeritus Professor of Healthcare Workforce Innovation.
2008

Preface

Veronica Bishop

The world today is changing at a tremendous speed; advances in technology and communication and changes in the political, economic, demographic and social changes, all touch our lives. These changes also impact on health care provision, and the delivery of health services. The aim of this book is to empower would – be leaders of nursing and allied health professions to be effective. Leadership in health care is a high priority in the UK and, at the time of writing, is top of the list for the National Health Service Federation. However, for nursing and those health care professions allied to medicine, leadership has rarely been a highly visible clear cut business. Certainly many consider that since the late 1990s, a severe erosion of power bases within the professions has occurred, particularly in the UK. There is no single reason for this – ownership of health care is now very diverse, with the traditional authority of medical colleagues restrained today by accountants, and to some extent by the blurring of professional boundaries – all of which is discussed in greater detail in the forthcoming chapters. While no patient wants a powerless professional taking care of them, nurses and allied health professionals (AHPs), who generally have the majority of patient contact, tend not to own any significant level of power in policymaking terms. Our professions have been caught in a web of strong threads which stem from such sources as gender stereotyping, medical dominance and inadequate professional leadership which conspire to keep us in the place where *others* would have us (Bishop 2002). To strengthen leadership within nursing and AHPs it is necessary to understand policy and professional contexts, and to review activities across Europe – now a growing entity – and the Atlantic. All health care professions ought to be playing a central role in making changes that will allow improvements in their health care system. Berwick (1994) considered that most proposed 'health reforms' made in Western society today were actually changes in the surroundings of care rather than changes in care itself. More recently Berwick (2003) suggests that for health professions to truly become involved requires a workforce capable of setting bold aims, measuring progress and finding alternative designs for the work itself. In so stating Berwick (2003) highlights the high degree of trust required to achieve this, and the necessary bias towards teamwork, as well as a predisposition to take the initiative in striving for improvement, rather than blaming external factors. This takes us to the core of what being a professional is, and in doing so we need to consider the role of a profession, and the obligation that accompanies that status. Thought-provoking issues arise here and are discussed at length in the text.

A major source of confusion and concomitant disappointment in relation to leadership is the lack of distinction between leadership and management. Disappointment arises because one often seems to negate the other, owing to lack of clarity of purpose. Bennis (1998), a prolific writer on the subject, suggests that we are under-led and over-managed. To contribute to new thinking on these two issues this publication unpicks, at some length, the differences between them, and offers a further concept for clinical health care staff to support clinical leadership. Here the importance of collaboration to achieve standards and quality, without loss of identity of one's discipline is discussed. And importantly, the core values that make working in health care a challenge well worth accepting are examined.

In looking afresh at leadership within the health care services and the necessary education to support that, the text includes a chapter that explores the impact of global health care reform and the changing role of the nurse, in order to concentrate on the implications of such radical and dynamic change on educating and developing the nurse leaders of the future. Complementary to this is a chapter on a programme devised to develop staff, enabling them to influence policy. This requires more than acquiring access to policymakers and using the right language; a set of skills and knowledge is needed that is not normally included in nurse training, and these are described in full, with case studies.

The book will be invaluable to:

- Students of nursing and health-related courses, at diploma and degree level.
- Educationalists teaching health care students of all disciplines, from diploma to postgraduate level.
- Managers and those on management courses.
- Clinical nurse specialists.
- Health care staff attending special courses in leadership.

If nurses and APHs are to maximize their contribution to health care, wherever they are in the world, there are important issues to be grasped. It is time for us to take stock, to promote and support our articulate and strategic thinkers, and to let them shine. This book will advance the understanding and significance of leadership in the health services, with the concomitant economic, political and social pressures. The following chapters will encourage understanding of the changing nature of leadership, putting into context current theories on leadership with case studies of past leadership figures. The ambiguities and complexities of leadership theory and practice are highlighted, and clear direction offered for the development of future leaders within a global health care context. Experts from a wide breadth of countries and knowledge have come together to help to achieve this.

References

Bennis, W. (1998) *Managing People is Like Herding Cats*. London: Kogan Page.

Berwick, D.M. (1994) Eleven worthy aims for clinical leadership of health system reform. *Journal of the American Medical Association* 272(10): 797–802.

Berwick, D.M. (2003) Improvement, trust and the health care workforce. *Quality and Safety in Health Care*. 12(6): 448–452.

Bishop, V. (2002) Editorial. *Journal of Research in Nursing* (formerly *Nursing Times Research*) 7(4): 240.

Introduction

Veronica Bishop

The grand old Duke of York, he had ten thousand men
He marched them up to the top of the hill
And he marched them down again.

(Traditional rhyme)

Leadership: why do we need it?

Leadership, or the need for it, appears to be inherent in the human make-up. This need may take various guises, as Bennis (1998) has noted, such as the idolization of successful sportsmen and women, the slavish adoration of glamorous film stars and pop singers. More focused leadership needs are evident in politics, in industry and in any group activity. Leadership is a way of focusing and motivating a group to enable them to achieve their aims. It also involves being accountable and responsible for the group as a whole. A leader should provide continuity and momentum, be flexible in allowing changes of direction, and ideally, a leader should be a few steps ahead of their team, but not too far for the team to be able to understand and follow them. Leadership is not just a person in a high position; to understand leadership we must also appreciate the interactions between a leader and his or her followers, and examine the dynamic nature of the relationship between leader and followers. Democracies elect leaders, small groups may select leaders, but however a leader is recognized, they are as dependent on their followers as the followers depend on them. Leaders are usually expected to provide a mutually beneficial vision for the way ahead, may take risks on their own and the group's behalf, and their term as a leader may be short lived or lengthy. There are many ambiguities surrounding the notion of leadership, but the first chapter aims to clarify the key issues that underpin leadership generally, before drawing the threads together to focus specifically on health care professionals.

World leaders: born of mothers or circumstance?

To understand leadership in the health care professions, it is helpful to 'step out of the box' and examine leadership as a worldwide phenomenon. One can too easily become enmeshed in micro politics of leadership, where one works, or even of one's country, without having a clear understanding of leadership in its entirety. Leadership is not a simple business! This book is one of hundreds, and many more will follow, each pursuing some angle of the concept of leadership. But for health care staff this one will, I hope, project thinking beyond the parochial and instil confidence in the reader to push a little at their boundaries, backed by an understanding of the very human issues involved.

The desire to follow a leader seems to be a common human instinct – less common is the ability to take on the leadership role. Why is this, and what makes one person raise their head above the parapet to be counted – or shot at? Two names come to mind who could have lived comfortable (and in one case luxurious lifestyles) if they had not done so; they are Winston Churchill and Osama Bin Laden. Churchill, born of powerful and weathly stock, writes in letters to his wife of knowing that he has a destiny (Soames 1999). I have no knowledge of Bin Laden having a notion of his destiny as a key player in world politics, but I do know that as an Arab prince of enormous wealth, he need not have been living in caves and shadows. His actions as a leader have impacted globally and will long outlive him. Both he and Churchill achieved global leadership status owing to political circumstances. How much does leadership depend on circumstance as much as characteristics?

It is undoubtedly a reflection of my age and interests, but asked to name a handful of world leaders, from across the ages, I would select Gandhi, Hitler (two very opposing philosophical approaches), Clinton, Thatcher and Queen Elizabeth I. This Queen must surely be one of the first women to break through the 'glass ceiling' of masculine domination – indeed her domination of men must appease the most ardent feminist! Boudicca may well have been as doughty but she did not, as far as my history takes me, start the change of England from an insignificant part of an island to a world player. Mahatma Gandhi, of course, was phenomenal, not only because of his intellect and wit, but also because of his adherence to the philosophy that peace was the only way to lasting victory, despite the very opposing views of both his enemies and his followers. And certainly, in his lifetime, he succeeded in realizing his ambition for India.

How different from my second selection – Adolf Hitler. But if we consider what a leader is – a person of dominance and persuasion who leads others for a period of time and, in the case of world politics, is widely noted, if not acclaimed – then Hitler fits the bill. Various dictators across the globe have come and gone, many of whom could reasonably be called evil, but few if any have the same resonance as Hitler. From the newer world there is Bill Clinton, twice elected president of the United States of America. A man of pleasant appearance and apparently huge charm, indeed a man, it seems, for all seasons and while infamous worldwide for a short time for behaving rashly privately and lying about it publicly, he remains famous today. Since he retired from office he has done, indeed still (at the time of writing) continues to carry out, works on a global scale in terms of charitable and ministerial missions. So do others, to name former United States President Jimmy Carter for one, but what of them? They appear to lack that elusive concept 'charisma' and thus go unremarked by the general population.

Margaret Thatcher, the first female prime minister of Great Britain, waved her handbag with a similar velocity to Queen Elizabeth ordering traitors to the Tower! Any glass ceiling here was quickly shattered, as were (in my personal view) many important social constructs within the United King-dom. However, this book is not about politics with a capital *P*, but the more potent politics (small *p*) of populations, their foci and their social and individual strategies for achieving what they deem to be beneficial to them. Did Margaret Thatcher have charisma? She certainly dominated with her presence and powerful men have admitted to finding her attractive. Watch-ing her many public appearances it always seemed to me that she bulldozed her way into the fore rather than being naturally blessed with charisma.

If I am allowed a sixth member in my handful – and in view of his outstanding contribution to our present world he cannot be left out – Nelson Mandela must surely count as a name that will resonate for many decades, if not centuries. His leadership through peaceful processes, seemingly devoid of bitterness despite 27 years of imprisonment for seeking rights for his people, his ambassadorship in negotiating the breakdown of apartheid with his one-time captors, make a spectacular study of leadership skills. In common with the selected case studies offered in this chapter, Mandela had a vision and never swerved from it. The skills to achieve such a vision will be studied in more depth in this book, as will the personalities of the previously mentioned leaders. Established theories of leadership will be examined in the light of these people.

Leadership in nursing: divide and overrule?

Leadership in the health services, and in nursing in particular, has a peculiar history. It is this peculiarity that has – especially in the case of nursing – lent

arid soil for growing and supporting leadership talent. Consider the begin-
nings of nursing, across the world. 'Wise' women, superstition, custom,
religion, nuns, sisters, and then the dragging of this unwieldy but essential
'apparatus' into education. Frame this collage within a male-dominated,
more educated authority, namely medicine, and then place the cold glass of
ever – changing politics and social funding across the whole picture. Davies
(2004) considers that a critical examination of the concept of political
leadership as it has recently developed in the field of nursing is needed. She
observes that to date the focus on political leadership is inward-looking and
individualizing, encouraging a view of the profession as immature and
disparate. Where nursing fits into current political health agendas today will
be considered in the final chapter, but Davies' astute doubts as to just how far
the historical neglect of nursing in policy areas has been overcome needs
careful consideration.

There has been a strong move from the United Kingdom government
since the late 1980s to reduce professional dominance in health care, with
considerable success. The mainly Thatcher-driven determination to reduce
the power of doctors had a significant knock-on effect on nursing. Nurses
have been lured with sweet words of teamwork and integrated working, as
well as higher salaries, away from patriarchal medical dominance into a
management hierarchy. Sadly, as I have commented elsewhere (Bishop 2005),
these structures often have little connection with patients and more in
common with Sainsbury's, a reflection on the fact that Thatcher pulled in a
chief executive of that supermarket to advise on health issues during her
time as prime minister! Many fine nurses suffered badly as a result of this
swift courtship, being cast off as soon as the next tranche of organizational
changes came along. Patriarchy possibly had a little more going for it. For
good or otherwise the general move of health care staff into teams, combined
with ever-changing needs of the public in response to new developments and
treatments, has blurred disciplinary boundaries.

This blurring is politically useful – the implications for the National
Health Service (NHS) workforce and the need to recruit staff, set against the
cost implications for mainly qualified staff, are enormous. Chronic shortages
of registered nurses, the majority of whom are female and many of whom are
bringing up young families or caring for elderly relatives, are compounded by
an ageing population, difficulties not confined to the UK as is to be learned
from Hanson and colleagues (2006). It must also be said that for some
individuals wonderful opportunities have been grasped, and dynamic ways
of providing services are evolving, but rarely within an overarching strategy,
and sometimes with very little collegiate support. At an international level
the work of the International Network for Doctoral Education in Nursing
(INDEN) aims to ameliorate this, impacting mainly in the academic sector
initially. An independent group, it is free to enter into partnership and

collaborative relationships internationally with other scholarly and professional groups of its choice for specific purposes in pursuit of its aims. Other examples of global collaboration among nurses can only hearten what sometimes seems to be an arid concept (for examples see *Journal of Research in Nursing* 2006 – vol 11.4).

My earlier view that the nursing profession is at a very important point in its development and one which requires careful consideration if it is not just to survive but to grow has not changed (Bishop 2005). 'Wrong footedness in the next few years will see the demise of a noble concept [of a nursing profession] (Bishop and Freshwater 2004: 196). Nursing lacks the coherence of other care disciplines – its positive strength in being fluid and responsive can too easily become a source of professional destruction. While other disciplines allied to medicine such as physiotherapy and radiography are often politically marginalized, mainly due to their smaller numbers, they do not lose their focus. Indeed inspiring examples are cited in Chapter 4 of how they have taken their clinical skills forward to meet new demands. Nursing, despite being the largest professional group in health care, seems to be caught in a web of strong threads which stem from such sources as gender stereotyping, medical dominance, political game playing, resource deprivation and inadequate professional leadership at many levels (Marriner 1994; Collinson 2002; Freshwater et al. 2002) which conspire to keep us in the place where others would have us.

Individuals can and do cut through some of this, but the real swathe cutting has to be highly visible at national and international levels. Nurses have a poor record of supporting each other, another reason why we have provided an easy target for those seeking to marginalize us. This is in part due to the fact that our history is hierarchical, and also because we do not have a culture of peer review, of critique and collegiate support. Clinical supervision was introduced in the early 1990s to change this, and is, slowly, being implemented across the UK, Scandinavia, Australia, New Zealand and the United States, but changing a culture takes decades (Bishop 2007). Despite many years of effort, the usual centrally led initiatives such as regional and national workshops and publicity through journals do not seem to be working effectively in the places where they are most needed. While time allocation set against funding is no small issue, there is still the apathy of a profession that is used to subjugation (see Chapter 3) and thus lacks the initiative to change. 'If you do what you always did, you get what you always got' – which in the case of all allied health professions (AHPs) is remarkably little. It is time for us to take stock, to promote and support our articulate and strategic thinkers, to let them shine.

As well as focusing on health care professionals in the UK, this book will argue that a new approach is needed to strengthen nursing leadership globally. Nurses in resource-rich countries need to support those in resource-poor settings without resorting to 'nursing imperialism'. The world is seeing a shift in economies with, particularly, China and India overtaking the established players in the world of finance and production. Communication is faster and easier than it has ever been and we cannot afford to merely focus parochially wherever we work, be it in Asia, the United States or the UK for example. This can seem very daunting for a single individual but it need not be if you really want to learn how to change things. The phrase 'one person can't make a difference' is not the mind-set of would-be leaders. Remember also that it is hard to change anything from the outside; you have to become involved, find out how to connect with what interests you. There are important structures existing that can be keyed into via the web, such as the International Council of Nurses (ICN), whose membership is drawn from formal nurse organizations across the world, and the World Health Organization (WHO), although this is a very medically led organization. Remember too Sigma Theta Tau (USA), whose vision is, through its members, to improve the health of the world's people. There are also many specialist group sites, such as cardiac care, urological nursing, and so on, with membership deriving from many countries.

It is important to remember that leadership is needed at every level of health care, particularly at the clinical level where nursing really counts. In the final chapter of this book, when the threads of all the contributions are pulled together, a strategy should be evolving in your mind that will help you focus on *your* leadership aspirations. This is a wake-up call to nurses everywhere to develop their leadership skills, and make a real difference to global health and social development. That is what this book is about.

References

Bennis, W. (1998) *Managing People is Like Herding Cats*. London: Kogan Page.

Bishop, V. (2005) Editorial. *Journal of Research in Nursing* 10(5): 485–486.

Bishop, V. (2007) Clinical supervision: What is it? Why do we need it? In V. Bishop (ed.) *Clinical Supervision in Practice: Some Questions, Answers and Guidelines for Professionals in Health and Social Care*. Basingstoke: Palgrave Macmillan.

Bishop, V. and Freshwater, D. (2004) Looking ahead: the future for nursing research. In D. Freshwater and V. Bishop (eds.) *Nursing Research in Context: Appreciation, Application and Professional Development*. Basingstoke: Palgrave Macmillan.

Collinson, G. (2002) The primacy of purpose and the leadership of nursing. *Nursing Times Research* (now *Journal of Research in Nursing*) 7(6): 403–411.

Davies, C. (2004) Political leadership and the politics of nursing. *Journal of Nursing Management* 12: 235–241.

Freshwater, D., Walsh, L. and Storey, L. (2002) Developing leadership through clinical supervision in prison health care. *Nursing Management*, 8(9): 16–20.

Hanson, E., Magnusson, L., Nolan, J. and Nolan, M. (2006) Developing a model of participatory research involving researchers, practitioners, older people and their family carers. *Journal of Research in Nursing* 11(4): 325–342.

Journal of Research in Nursing (2006) Focus: International collaboration – Sharing lessons learned. 11(4).

Marriner, A.C. (1994) Theories of leadership. In C.E. Hein and M.J. Nicholson (eds) *Contemporary Leadership Behavior*, 4th edn. Philadelphia, PA: Lippincott.

Soames, M. (ed.) (1999) *Speaking for Themselves*. London: Transworld, Random House.

(1) What is leadership?

Veronica Bishop

Overview

Central to this chapter is the deconstruction of leadership itself, citing world famous leaders and global influences. Focusing then on the allied health care professionals, the historic, political and gender impact on these professions is highlighted. Particular attention is paid to nursing as the largest NHS group of employees, and its power bases are examined, focusing particularly on the period since 1988. In considering where nursing has come from, the shape of the profession, the nature of the work and the value placed on it, questions are raised as to how it might consider its place in the future.

Setting the scene: why is professional leadership needed in health care settings?

It could be argued that to promote powerful leadership in all the allied health disciplines within an already heavily managed system is unlikely to achieve anything but turf wars; indeed historically this has more often than not been the case. At the inception of health care programmes within the Western world, there was something to be said for a more hierarchical system, where each knew their place. Saks, in Chapter 3, succinctly describes the perceived vulnerability of physicians in the early days of organized health care in Western society, and their very successful manoeuvres to establish professional dominance in pursuance of self-interest. In health care today it is unlikely that such elitist tactics would appeal to, or be upheld by, any professional group for any length of time. Medical dominance no longer remains socially appropriate (if it ever was) but is in fact unworkable in today's society where professionals have their own codes of practice and must fit their contribution to care within the jigsaw of a complete care programme that seeks to meet the demands of a rising consumer movement. We are now accustomed to collaborative working, are in many cases as well educated as our professional neighbours, and are well aware of global economies and their impact on health care resources. However, increased diversity, individualization and consumerism have led to a far more complex view of health both by the public and by health professionals (Wilmot 2003).

Health care is an economically as well as socially driven phenomenon, there are vested interests throughout and attempts to claim 'ground' from a range of interested parties. Not only have small societies such as professional groups been sorely challenged by these complexities, but also the impact of changes within greater global communities is felt locally, a view supported by Bottery (1998). Major events such as the breaking up of Russia, the growing power of China and India, and the growth of groups such as the United Nations and the European Community affect us all, not least as they are underpinned by a preference by most governments of almost all philosophies, to run with the apparent superiority of free market logic. Margaret Thatcher, UK prime minister from 1979 until 1990, embraced this wholeheartedly, introducing an internal market (that is a quasi-market in health care in which the state provides the finances but in which competition exists between independent suppliers to provide the service) within the NHS, and establishing a central tenet that health was to be run as a business. Despite Thatcher's fall from grace, and the election of a supposedly socialist Labour government in 1997, the basic philosophy has not changed, and the effect of all this for many has been a slow but insidious erosion of those core values of caring that drew many professionals into health care in the first place. Bottery (1998) noted from his research in the UK that professionals who had seen themselves as principal contributors to a co-ordinated system for the greater public good now perceive themselves as being mere functionaries of a system that resembles a marketplace that rates economy, efficiency and effectiveness above all else. That resources cannot be unlimited, that accountability for those resources must be made, is unquestioned by most health care staff. Indeed, on the face of it the values of evidence-based effectiveness would not cause health professionals any anxiety. However, strong policy interests are apt to dominate the judgements made in the name of evidence – based health care. Given the quasi-market values of policymakers and senior management, health care workers are finding that their practice is moulded into that culture, presenting them with ethical and legislative challenges (Bottery 1998). Ethical issues such as the promotion of policies that are narrow (for example Murray et al. 2008), lack of properly qualified staff for the provision of safe care (Buchan 2002, 2004) and the obligation to pursue inadequately funded or poorly thought out strategies (Bottery 1998).

It is the response of health professionals to the changes described above that will set the scene, indeed write the script, for future decades of health care services. Despite the fact that collaboration between health disciplines is now commonplace in Western society, and the balance of power has shifted slightly from medical dominance to a more shared philosophy, none of the health care professionals – including doctors – have real ownership of the care that they provide. Public health care is owned by the funding governments, and as such, those professionals participating in its function such as doctors, nurses and therapists must – to have an effective voice – be cohesive.

Robinson (1992) blamed competing groups within nursing for failing to set occupational objectives within the wider socio-economic context of health, and attributed nursing's subordination to its own divisiveness, a point expanded on by Stanley in Chapter 2. Certainly today's health care professionals need to consider the nature of their role within society as a whole, not just within their organization. Only by reflecting on their professional function in its entirety can new ways of effective working become established. This move from a tightly marginalized group to a cohesive and collaborative workforce requires clarity of vision, a wide breadth of knowledge, and strong leadership. In countries where patriarchy dominates, lessons may be learned from current developments in Hong Kong in particular, and from some understanding of how Western societies have moved on to some degree. In health care this has taken longer than in many other groupings and explanations of why are well described by Saks in Chapter 3.

Leadership characteristics: inherited or learned trait?

Leadership, even in democracies, is central to the functioning of most societies, and involves at least two people in pursuit of a common goal. The literature identifies leadership as one of the critical success factors for sustaining continuous improvement in any organization (Zairi 1994; Taffinder 1995). Health disciplines working under the umbrella of one organization need, for optimum functioning, to be very clear as to the aims of that organization and – most importantly – they must also have clarity about their professional role and contribution to the business of health care. This clarity can come only from good leadership, at both national and local levels.

Bennis (1998 p. 161) considers that the need for leaders currently goes unspoken, while being 'pathetically' manifest in our idolatry of show business stars. He also notes that leadership courses are consuming billions of dollars with little sign of any leaders. So what is leadership? Stogdill (1974) wrote that there are almost as many definitions of leadership as people who have tried to define it, and in the intervening decades this is still true. It is important to differentiate, at the outset of this chapter, between great people and leaders. Scientists, heroes, Nobel prize-winners and wonderful individuals may or may not become leaders in the general understanding of the word, and some very sinister or intellectually challenged people can join the ranks of leaders. Leaders can give hope and direction or turn the world upside down; how they have such power is what we must begin to examine.

Leadership theories have developed from Machiavelli (1532), whose observations of the powerful Borgias who ruled while he served in Florence are written for posterity in *Il Principe* (*The Prince*). In his writings he noted the importance of shared information between those with power and influence, and the need for courtesy between collaborating parties. Today he is mainly identified with the adjective 'Machiavellian' meaning cunning or devious, owing to his theory that the end justifies the means. Girvin (1998) cites Galton (1870) as a relatively more recent contributor to leadership theory, with his perception of the heroic; a leader of troops with inherited characteristics of leadership, qualities passed down through generations. To some degree this view holds today, with wealthy families creating dynasties, and public (so called, but expensive and private) schools such as Eton in England being viewed as the most suitable institutions for educating and instilling leadership qualities in youngsters.

Max Weber (1864–1920), founder of modern sociological thought and cited in more depth by Saks in Chapter 3, took the debate further by defining three key bases for leadership power, described by Smith and Peterson (1988, cited by Girvin 1998):

- The *rational base*, which assumed the prevailing social norm as correct and that those in authority had the right to command.
- The *traditional base*, where the belief in a traditional power and authority holds.
- The *charismatic base*, where an individual possessing particular characteristics is given power.

Interestingly, it was Weber (1947) who introduced the term 'charisma', which (literally translated from Greek) means gift of grace. Frank (1993) posits that in essence this means that the person has the ability to develop or inspire others in an ideological commitment to a particular point of view. There are those, for example Roberts (2004), who consider that comparisons may be drawn between true inspiration and 'mere' charisma. Roberts cites comparisons between Hitler and Churchill, two world leaders who were in forceful opposition. He finds Hitler charismatic and Churchill truly inspirational. I would suggest that this is a value judgement based on the atrocities carried out in Hitler's name rather than a clear-cut rationale. Inspirational or not, when the British public no longer felt a need for Churchill's brand of leadership they dropped him – his earlier triumphs a thing of the past, suggesting that even inspiration may be a transient talent. Charisma is often evident by a person's presence or attractiveness combined with a positive and engaging manner. Conveying by a confident voice and positive eye contact that whomever you are talking to matters can be learned, as can good posture and the development of a wardrobe that gives you confidence. Charismatic people have sparkle, indicating an energy that their audience finds motivating, and while some people seem to be charismatic naturally, it can be learned, developed and honed as long as it is done with sincerity. Otherwise it will fail horribly!

Fundamentally, as Bennis (1998: 3) states, the key attributes of successful leaders are quite clear. They are 'people who are able to express themselves fully … they know what they want and how to communicate what they want to other people in order to gain their co-operation and support'. Subsequent numerous studies on leadership following Weber's earlier work cited above have resulted in a highly sophisticated set of interconnected views on leadership. I have concertinaed them into four, as the differences between some are subtle to the point of confusion. None are clear-cut as one theory may overlap with another, but the categorization allows distinctions to be made between genetic, circumstantial and learned styles of leadership.

1   (Genetic) Great man theory – leadership is inherent, not made. Based on military leadership concepts; traditional power bases of dynasties, and inherited genes.
    Examples: Ruling families, nobility, feudal kingdoms, family businesses.

2   (Genetic or learned) Trait theory, charisma – assumes qualities of persuasion, which can be inherited or developed.
    Examples: Individuals who attract followers.

3   (Circumstantial) Contingency and situational theories – environmental factors determining style of leadership; this leadership may be transient.
    Examples: Someone who takes control and holds the group's confidence, for example in a shipwreck.

4   (Circumstantial or learned) Behavioural and participation theories – defined by actions, not genes. These include:

● (Learned) Transactional theory – based on a system of reward and punishment, e.g. *Management systems* (*see Chapter 2*).

● (Charismatic or learned) Transformational theory – based on motivating and inspiring others, e.g. *the moving of followers beyond their self-interest for the good of the group, organization, or society.*

While leadership is central to the survival of most groups and organizations, the style of leadership depends on external factors and must fit with the environment of the time – even charismatic leaders may have a limited leadership span.

For those readers wishing to access a substantive and quite recent review of leadership studies, I recommend the work of Osseo-Asare et al. (2005), which looks at best practice in leadership in higher education. In this work leadership was found to be one of the critical success factors for sustaining quality and performance improvement in United Kingdom higher education institutions. Results also indicated that leadership ought to be effectively integrated with policy and strategy, and deliberately exercised through process ownership and improvement. Of course environmental issues impact on an individual's responses; many people may have the characteristics seen as essential for an effective leader but are never in a situation to call them into play. Further, the great man or trait theory may be restrained by environmental factors, so the notion of one wrap-around theory is as far removed today as it was in Machiavelli's time. To add to this lack of absolute clarity is the fusion, or confusion, between management and leadership. This is a crucial issue for health care professionals that is considered in depth by Stanley in Chapter 2. Suffice to say, in sympathy with Bennis's view that today we are 'over-managed and under-led' (Bennis 1998: 161), and for the purposes of this chapter, I will focus on the emotional rather than the functional aspect of leadership.

Bennis (1997) considers that a leader is more than the sum of his or her parts, and makes more of their experiences. He lists leadership qualities as:

● Integrity
● Dedication
● Magnanimity
● Openness
● Creativity
● Optimism
● Risk taking
● Passion.

His portrait of a leader is a person with self-knowledge, a strongly defined sense of purpose, the capacity to generate and sustain trust and to have a bias towards action. Bennis totally refutes the notion of born leaders, considering leadership to be learned through life and work experiences. This is consistent with the work of Osseo-Asare et al. (2005) where some respondents confirmed that they exercised leadership on the basis of what Mullins (1999) described as 'sapiential authority', that is by wisdom, personal knowledge, and reputation or expertise. Gardner (1989) studied a large number of North American organizations and leaders, and came to the conclusion that there were some qualities or attributes that enabled a leader in one situation to lead in another. These range from vitality and stamina to 'people skills', competence and courage. In my view Bennis hits the nail when he speaks of passion. It is passion that fuels an individual to realize their vision; passion that provides the energy, but this is not enough without a power base, and this was never more true than in the health services.

Power

Leadership without power is of little use in any environment; however, power is a concept that not everyone is comfortable with. It appears to go against our notions of democracy and equality. Nonetheless without a power base little can be accomplished outside the norm. An oft-quoted study that demonstrates this well is that carried out by Lewin et al. (1939). In their study of groups of youngsters it was noted that those following a democratic style of leadership got along together but did not accomplish difficult tasks so well, while those under a more authoritarian leadership style achieved more. Those with a laissez-faire approach were unsupportive to each other and accomplished little.

Central to leadership in health care is the notion of mastery. Mastery is an acquired set of competencies that provides a baseline of knowledge and expertise for a leader. With mastery comes a level of self-confidence in what the leader brings to the table. To be involved in health care, mastery of expert practice in a specialty or generalist area is often a stepping stone to becoming a leader, be it at a local level or at a wider forum such as a speciality network, or organization. The confidence that is derived from developing mastery can be empowering, and power is essential to leadership. Knowledge is intellectual power, credibility among peers. However, most of us will have met very knowledgeable individuals who fail to communicate or inspire others around them – they work well but have no shared vision; change is not on their agenda. *Leaders are marked by their desire to meet challenges, to move forward, and to do this they use their knowledge and extend their private world to embrace those around them.* While power bases come from varying sources, the most common types fall into one of three categories:

- Informational power

- Authoritarian power
- Charismatic power.

Informational power

Informational power is not only having knowledge but also using it creatively and politically. This involves an ability to connect and to relate to
others and begins to address the issue of inspiring others. Nurses have more
information about patients, their families and communities than any other
professional group, yet nurses tend to be unaware and unable to own any
significant level of power. No patient wants a powerless health professional.

Authoritarian power

Positions of authority carry an expectation of power, 'legitimate power',
which is hierarchical in its principles. The history of allied health professionals to medicine is rooted in this tradition of leadership and power. Despite
the fact that nursing in the UK has moved from the patriarchy of medicine, it
has not yet stood alone as a professional entity but has borrowed the mantle
of management and legitimized a fragile power base often away from clinical
work, an issue picked up in Chapters 2 and 7 by Stanley in his work on
cognitive leadership. While there are some moves to relocate a clinical power
base for nurses, that power is, in the UK at least, more aligned to very
specialized areas rather than across the board. Power bases for therapists,
discussed fully in Chapter 4, are more likely to develop from their clinical
area of expertise.

Charismatic power

A third type of power is known as charismatic. Put simply, this is power
derived from charm or personality. Charm may be 'turned on' but is none
the less real, and can move and inspire huge crowds or just one other
individual. The essence of charm is to enchant and to be believable.
Charismatic people are usually great orators, motivating those around them
and inspiring greater determination. While the power of fine speaking gives
them a head start in the leadership stakes, oration on its own is not enough.
The warmth that comes from caring about people and letting it show, by
being positive and portraying a goal that is achievable and can be shared,
and – most importantly – valuing the contribution made by those that are
being led, lends real fire to the charismatic. Girvin (1998) notes that

personality power can too easily be abused, and the historical case studies described later in this chapter will demonstrate the truth of this!

None of these power bases are mutually exclusive, and a major task for any leader is to hold diverse parts of a system, conflicting issues among teams, and opposing arguments from equally worthy professional groups.

Historical perspectives: selected case studies

Leadership qualities are not specific to one environment. Leaders in health care will have the same attributes as leaders of huge conglomerates, successful businesses and charitable organizations, or educational institutions for example. To consider leadership qualities let us take well-known examples of leaders from across the world. Within the confines of one part of one book it is neither possible, nor necessarily helpful, to delve deeply into historical analysis, but a brief historical perspective may be very helpful in matching current theories of leadership to some well-known leaders. Thumbnail sketches may offend academic historians but for our purposes they can be very useful and illustrative. Moving in chronological order to consider the handful of well-documented leaders that I selected in the Introduction, we will consider a brief history of each.

Queen Elizabeth I of England (1533–1603)

Elizabeth was the daughter of King Henry VIII and his second wife, Anne Boleyn. He had desperately hoped for a son to succeed him as he already had a daughter by his first wife. Elizabeth's early life was consequently troubled, not least by the execution of her mother and the declaration that her mother's marriage to the king was null and void. Declared illegitimate and deprived of her place in the line of succession, the next eight years of her life saw a quick succession of stepmothers. Here was a woman of highest rank but whose security was, in her youth, very fragile, given that the beheading of inconvenient royals was not uncommon then and she was, for some time, perceived as very inconvenient. Her father sired one legitimate son, Edward VI, who was crowned king but died at the age of 15 years. Despite a troubled accession to the throne, her good education combined with her natural intelligence, eventually led her to becoming a sovereign of great significance, taking England, which had been racked by religious wars and poverty, to relative peace and considerable riches. Her reign is often referred to as 'The Golden Age' of English history. She was an immensely popular queen, and her popularity has waned little with the passing of time. Testimony to this are the frequent cinematic portrayals of her life. She became a legend in her own lifetime, famed for her remarkable abilities and achievements.

- Her leadership skills are best described as somewhat Machiavellian, as she played prospective suitors along while never conceding to their wishes, but all the while strengthening her position. Her leadership stemmed from the rational and traditional, with a style that was typical of the day, autocratic and transactional (punishment/reward). Her power base derived from being the greatest power in the land, with all the coercion that meant in those days! None the less, many profited by her rule, and there was little attempt to remove her from the throne once her inherent strengths became obvious.

Gandhi (1869–1948)

Gandhi was born in India into a family of high caste (status), and his father held a leadership position in the area, so the notion of being born into a leadership role has a bearing here. Despite being a shy and mediocre student both at school and at college, he went to England to study to be a barrister, where he was very homesick. Immediately after passing his examinations he enrolled at the High Court in London and promptly sailed home the next day. Two years later, having had little success in establishing a law firm in Bombay, he joined an Indian firm with interests in South Africa and went to their Durban office as a legal adviser. Shocked by the widespread denial of civil liberties and political rights to Indian immigrants there, he threw himself into the struggle for their elementary rights, remaining there for 20 years and suffering imprisonment many times. In 1914 the government of the Union of South Africa made important concessions to Gandhi's demands, including recognition of Indian marriages and abolition of the poll tax for them.

His work in South Africa complete, he returned to India where he became the most prominent leader in a complex struggle with Britain and fellow Indians for Indian home rule. Becoming the international symbol of a free India, he lived a spiritual and ascetic life of prayer, fasting and meditation. Periods of imprisonment for civil non-compliance met by fasting and peaceful non-co-operation served to strengthen his standing with his countrymen, who revered him as a saint and began to call him Mahatma (great-souled), a title reserved for the greatest sages. Gandhi's advocacy of non-violence is implicit in the Hindu religion, and it was through his adherence to this that Britain eventually realized that violence here was futile and gave India its freedom, although his triumph was tempered by disappointment at the partition of India. Gandhi's assassination was regarded as an international catastrophe, and his place in humanity was measured not in terms of the twentieth century, but in terms of history. A period of mourning was set aside in the United Nations General Assembly, and condolences to India were expressed by all countries.

- Here we have a classic example of a visionary who responded to environmental and contingency issues, moved by a powerful sense of what is right. To say that Gandhi did not use coercion would not be strictly true – threatening to starve yourself to death if change is not achieved must be regarded as coercive, and the use of self rather than arms or violence indicates an acute awareness of one's worth. That surely was his power base, the knowledge of his influence on others around him. Biographies portray a man of great wit, a seeker of truth and a philosopher whose life might have been quietly spent meditating rather than challenging the most powerful politicians of the time.

Adolf Hitler (1889–1945)

Hitler has had more biographies written about him than any other world leader and while he must be held accountable for millions of lost and tortured lives, I suspect that this is not the only reason for such exposure. He just does not present a profile, initially, of a world leader, and there, I suspect, lies the fascination for biography writers.

He grew up with a poor record at school and left, before completing his tuition, with a vague ambition to become an artist. His father died when Hitler was 13 and between the ages of 16 and 19 he neither worked nor studied, but developed an interest in politics and history. At 19, after the death of his mother, he moved to Vienna in the hope of earning a living. However, within a year he was living in homeless shelters and eating at charity soup-kitchens; at this time the German economy was in dire straits and Hitler developed a hatred for non-Germans. At the outbreak of the First World War in 1914, he volunteered for service but despite being decorated rose only to corporal level. While working for a local army organization his ability to deliver fiery and eloquent speeches was noted and he was given responsibility for publicity and propaganda. Here he honed his oratory skills, and after the war he joined the National Socialist German Workers Party, known as the Nazis, later becoming its leader and increasing its membership quickly with his powerful speeches. Following a failed attempt to storm the government, Hitler was arrested and sentenced to prison where he laid out his vision for Germany in *Mein Kampf* (*My Struggle*). Released after nine months, he began to rebuild the Nazi Party and in 1933 he was appointed Chancellor of Germany. From this position Hitler moved quickly toward attaining a dictatorship. Under his government there was no place for freedom; the government controlled every part of people's lives. Hitler used extensive propaganda to brainwash the nation into believing his theory about creating the perfect Aryan race. The atrocities and millions killed that were carried out to achieve this 'perfection' are fully documented elsewhere and still torment us today.

- Here was a man of insignificant stature, from an equally insignificant background, with little education. How could such a person lead a disparate population and almost win Europe? He is portrayed as immensely charismatic, not given to detail but preferring to leave that to others, and with an ability to orate and stir the masses. Circumstances in Germany at that time were dire; if they had not been, how differently might history have been written? Would his vision combined with his oratory skills have moved so many so far from decency? His introduction to power was his oratory, his later more 'coercive' tactics enabled him to hold on to it. The lesson here could be 'beware of charisma'!

Nelson Mandela (1918–)

Mandela was born in South Africa, the child of a chieftain. Despite his mother being one of the less important wives, Mandela received a good education, as well as a taste for rebellion, participating in student protests against apartheid. After qualifying in law he joined the African National Congress (ANC). When the ANC was banned in 1960, Mandela engaged in active military resistance against the ruling National Party's apartheid policies, resulting in him being brought to stand trial for plotting to overthrow the government by violence. He refused legal representation in court and his statement from the dock received considerable international publicity. Nevertheless he was sentenced to life imprisonment.

During his years in prison, where he studied assiduously, his reputation grew steadily, and he was widely accepted as the most significant black leader in South Africa. He became a potent symbol of resistance as the anti-apartheid movement gathered strength, and consistently refused to compromise his political position to obtain his freedom. Despite being removed from society he had become a huge thorn in the flesh of the ruling white class. While imprisoned his philosophy changed from a militant approach, to one that valued peaceful processes, and from prison he initiated a peaceful transition to a more democratic country. When he was released in 1990, after 27 years in prison, he plunged himself wholeheartedly into his life's work, striving to attain the goals, through peaceful means, that he and others had set out almost four decades earlier. His leadership skills were now to become crucial to achieve his vision. He had to win the support of his followers and allay the fears of the ruling white population.

In 1991, at the first national conference of the ANC held inside South Africa after the organization had been banned in 1960, Mandela was elected its president. He and F.W. de Klerk, the then South African white president, worked together to end apartheid and to bring about a peaceful transition to non-racial democracy in South Africa. In 1993 they shared the Nobel Prize for Peace for their efforts. The patience, wisdom and visionary quality that he brought to his struggle, and above all the moral integrity with which he set about to unify a divided people, resulted in the country's first democratic elections and his selection as president. He was inaugurated as the first democratically elected State President of South Africa in May 1994 and served until June 1999. Mandela has received numerous prestigious awards, and at the time of writing is a revered world leader. While he has retired from official work he is greatly sought after to endorse the work of others – a gold-plated sign of validity!

- Mandela considered that he was an ordinary man who became a leader because of extraordinary circumstances. Nonetheless we must recall that he came from a leading family in his area thus was possibly not uncomfortable with a leadership role. This is similar to the circumstances of both Gandhi and Thatcher. In common with them he had a firm and unshakeable vision, and the intellect to facilitate it. Knowledge brought him power and combined with his passion he was able to 'sell' his vision. That he has the common touch and is charismatic comes over clearly on all media coverage of him, and while he is a South African, born and bred, the entire world embraces him as theirs.

Margaret Thatcher (1925–)

Margaret Thatcher is considered by many to be the most significant English-woman since Elizabeth I, and was the first woman to head the government of one of the major world economies. Born in Grantham where her father ran a grocer's shop and served as a senior member of the city, Thatcher was academically bright and went to Oxford University to study chemistry and law. Interested in politics she was elected, aged 34, to Parliament, where she rose to ministerial level as Secretary of State for Education – a position often given to a woman, and usually as far as a female could expect to get in a UK government. In a challenge for the Conservative Party leadership she became, unexpectedly, its first female leader. During her premiership unem-ployment rose steeply but her conviction that a tight economy would bring future benefits was very persuasive, and she remained in power. This was greatly helped by the enormous patriotic enthusiasm that followed her successful repulsion of the invasion by Argentina of the British-owned

Falkland Islands. This euphoria was enhanced by a uselessly divided opposition; Thatcher secured three consecutive general elections, a rare achievement. A champion of free markets and capitalism she introduced a system of an internal market into the NHS (see page 9), which was to place management in the highest position in the national health care system – still evident to date. Perhaps more to her credit was her concern on environmental issues voiced in the late 1980s when she made a major speech accepting the problems of global warming, ozone depletion and acid rain. Thatcher stated that she owed nothing to feminism; it could also be said that she did nothing for it. As the wife of a wealthy and supportive man she was able to work and run a family of two children with comparative ease. She was a tireless worker famously requiring little more than four hours sleep a night, and totally committed to her work. Aware of the massive impact of the media, particularly television, her voice, once somewhat tedious, was trained to more modulated tones, and her hair and clothes were 'made over' to promote an acceptable image – with considerable success.

Margaret Thatcher, like Elizabeth I, was apt to surround herself with young men, and women were not encouraged into her cabinet. Indeed the one woman who did achieve notable cabinet status (Edwina Currie) was dropped as soon as her profile became competitive. Apparently many men found the so-called 'Iron Lady' attractive, but increasingly her autocratic approach lost her a great deal of support. Her characteristics were profoundly warrior-like, and while apparently in private she was capable of changing her mind with bewildering speed, once set on a course she would not change her opinion nor listen to others with differing views. This strength of character that had taken her from the back benches to the fore was, in the end, to be her destruction. Widespread opposition to poll tax (community charge) culminated in a huge demonstration in 1990 in London that turned into the largest outbreak of public disorder that the UK capital had seen in a century. This, combined with her government's proposed policy on entry into Europe, which was ill-timed economically, and her perceived arrogance made her vulnerable. Her Chancellor resigned, igniting a leadership challenge which resulted in an unsustainable narrow win. Thatcher resigned, leaving her admirers and critics to scrabble among themselves to find a new leader.

- Margaret Thatcher, like Gandhi and Mandela, was born into a family that held some position in its locality, and they also shared a personal conviction that theirs was the way forward – they had a vision. The word charisma is rarely used for Thatcher, the force rather than the charm of her personality was noted. Her power base was authoritative – the given right of a party leader and later, a premier – but she lacked what is known as 'the common touch', maintaining an autocratic approach which undoubtedly contributed to her downfall.

Bill Clinton (1946–)

The 42nd president of the United States of America, Clinton was born three months after his father died in a road accident, and took the name of his alcoholic and abusive car salesman stepfather when he was 14. Clinton proved to be an able student and a good musician. Graduating from university he won a Rhodes Scholarship to Oxford University and received a law degree from Yale University in 1973. He entered politics in Arkansas and became president in 1993, serving until 2001. During his administration Clinton defied his critics by surviving an array of personal scandals that the media highlighted across the world, and by sidestepping many major issues such as global warming. Despite this he turned the greatest fiscal deficit in American history into a surplus, achieving the lowest unemployment rate in modern times, the highest home ownership in the country's history, and lowest crime rates in many places, with reduced welfare rolls. His influence was not restricted to home and he effectively used American force to stop the murderous 'ethnic cleansing' wars in Bosnia and Kosovo. His popularity was such that he was the first Democratic president since Franklin D. Roosevelt to win a second term. As part of a plan to celebrate the millennium in 2000, Clinton called for a great national initiative to end racial discrimination, and has been described as the first 'black' president in the United States. After the failure in his second year of a huge programme of health care reform, Clinton shifted emphasis and sought legislation to upgrade education, to protect jobs of parents who must care for sick children, to restrict handgun sales, and to strengthen environmental rules.

Following the end of his presidency Clinton has remained very involved in global initiatives through his Foundation. This was formed to strengthen the capacity of people throughout the world to meet the challenges of global interdependence, working principally through partnerships with like-minded individuals, organizations, corporations and governments, often serving as a sounding board for new policies and programmes. Clinton is the typical charismatic leader, creating empathy with his audiences and projecting a deep concern for their welfare.

- My exposure to both Margaret Thatcher and to Bill Clinton has been solely through the media, television in particular. That Clinton is widely acknowledged as attractive is only part of the reason that I can recall his personality so well: he has huge charisma, and this comes through when people talk of meeting with him and when you hear him speak it is difficult to doubt his sincerity. Unlike Hitler, he has used his charisma very differently – though not without indiscretion – and is, at the time of writing nearly a decade after his presidency, still an enormously popular international figure.

Power bases in health care today

The creation of the National Health Service in the United Kingdom in 1948, offering free health care at the point of delivery financed by general taxation, was a remarkable achievement that has been the envy of many countries and has served as a model system. The dominant biomedical model of health care that underpinned its introduction has predominated for most of the twentieth century. Much of the rationale for this is discussed fully in Chapter 3, with fascinating insights of similarities on both sides of the Atlantic, and with doctors holding the reins of power. However, the ever-increasing cost of the NHS has always made it an obvious political football, and one which prime minister Margaret Thatcher kicked firmly into play, bringing together earlier moves to introduce management structures via the Griffiths Report (Department of Health and Social Security (DHSS 1983) that significantly restrained the authority of doctors. This was not without a knock-on effect, causing Robinson to note that 'nursing after Griffiths has lost any illusion of the power it might have once possessed' (Robinson 1992: 3). In fact the power base of nursing before the Griffiths management structures were implemented was very much a patriarchal one gifted from medical colleagues, rather than a true power base. While little has changed in the balances of power within health care disciplines since the creation of the NHS, a combination of many factors including increased diversity of health care options, increased emphasis on health education and promotion, the more open promotion of alternative therapies and a more aware, and litigious society and accompanying raised 'user' power has effected more opportunity for change than any single government.

In the 1990s nurse education in the UK moved from hospital-based schools of nursing into institutes of higher education, with the awarding of qualifications that were academically meaningful. At the same time junior doctors' hours were being reduced to less arduous levels, and these two changes are unlikely to be unrelated! Nurses were to take on more work. Those nurses who had been quietly specializing in a given clinical area began to flourish openly, becoming consultants or advanced practitioners. This should have been advantageous to the profession as a whole, and in some cases it is, but as Stanley reports in Chapter 7, often these new posts have a high management content and are often seen as divisive. At the same time that the new UK structures of acute health services were being introduced there was a legal obligation to include a nurse at board level, thus appearing to improve the status of nurses and other related health care professionals. Nursing, a discipline that has its history rooted in male-dominated hierarchical systems (initially the church and later medicine), rose to the management challenge with what could be seen, with hindsight, as thoughtless enthusiasm. For despite this apparent entrée into health care politics, many management courses later, and the International Council of Nurses (ICN 2001) moves to improve nurses' political and leadership expertise, nurses in all countries of the world continue to experience difficulties accessing and influencing local, national and international political agendas (Hennessy 2000; West and Scott 2000; Maslin-Prothero and Masterson 2002; Antrobus 2003). The reasons for this are discussed more fully in Chapter 5 and constructive ways forward offered.

There are important lessons here for those countries that are moving towards the UK model, such as India and China. In India, colleges of nursing, offering diploma and degree courses, are expanding in number, while China has been strongly influenced by long-running developments in Hong Kong, where there have been major developments in nursing practice and education since the mid 1990s. In 1995 nursing education in Hong Kong moved into higher education and a four-year honours degree programme became the major route for pre-registration nursing education. Postgraduate education has also developed rapidly following the introduction of the first taught Master of Nursing programme at the Chinese University of Hong Kong in 1995. Master of Nursing programmes are now offered in an increasing number of specialities, with a significant number of nurses going on to complete doctoral studies. Although some universities are offering a choice of taught doctoral programmes based on the USA model, the majority of doctoral programmes are research based drawing on the UK model. It is perhaps of note that all academic staff working with nursing programmes in Hong Kong universities are required to hold a doctoral degree for posts of assistant professor and above, prior to taking up their appointment – a practice that has not been implemented widely in the UK. A similar expansion of education programmes has taken place in mainland China, with figures suggesting a total of 179 undergraduate programmes in 2005. Although some universities now offer taught Master of Nursing programmes, nurses in mainland China wishing to complete PhD programmes are currently receiving their education mainly in the United States or Hong Kong. The growth of postgraduate programmes has led to a major increase in research activity particularly in Hong Kong and currently all academic staff in Hong Kong are expected to be research active.

Nursing practice has also developed rapidly since the late 1990s in Hong Kong with developments that have involved the implementation of clinical nurse specialist posts, advanced practice roles such as nurse-led clinics and most recently piloting of nurse consultants. Interestingly, the location of Hong Kong means that nursing developments have been influenced by US, UK and Australian models of care. For example a nurse practitioner programme based on the US model has been implemented, although difficulty has been experienced in obtaining the 500 required clinical hours and appropriate mentors for clinical practice (difficulties that are not uncommon in the UK). The nurse consultant model is being developed from the UK model bringing an eclectic approach to nurse development and leadership. Generally, however, developments have focused on advanced practice roles, linked to the Master's programmes and nurses usually require a Master's degree to take on the role of an advanced practice nurse. An Academy of Nursing is currently being developed to accredit specialization in nursing and to facilitate the development of expertise in advanced practice. In mainland China the increasing contact between nurses and academic staff in Hong Kong has contributed to the early developments of advanced practice roles in mainland China. These moves to improve care and develop expertise must be praised, but those leaders involved with these new developments may care to heed the work of Stevens (1997: 10), who noted that 'the art is in recognising the need for specialisation but not allowing it to become segregation or professional insularity, potentially leading it to oblivion.'

One issue that still has to be considered in China on the development of advanced practice is that of nurse prescribing. Currently nurses do not have the right to prescribe, which is constraining the development of some nurse-led roles. Current anecdotal evidence suggests there is reluctance among medical practitioners and pharmacists for nurses to take on such roles (Twinn 2008, personal communication). While in the UK nurse prescribing and the role of the nurse practitioner has moved on, albeit slowly, it is in management structures that any real professional power exists. Interestingly, our medical colleagues rarely drop their medical expertise entirely in exchange for a management post, whereas nurses do. There is a strongly held view that the continued move to integrate nursing into a general management framework has resulted in further marginalization of nursing leadership and has served the nursing profession badly, a view highlighted by Greer (2004). While devolution has brought interesting changes in this area and while there is evidence of professional coherence in Scotland, Northern Ireland and Wales, Greer's observations are less positive about England. He observes that the most visible experiments in health policy have been carried out in England, but comments on the restlessness and often heedlessness of these exercises. The resultant lack of cohesion and somewhat opportunistic approach to health care has had a profound effect on nurse leadership in England, and there is a view that the nursing profession in the UK generally has never been more vulnerable than it is at present.

The reasons for this are not difficult to identify. In recent years no one has consolidated the attention of the nursing profession in the UK, and maintained that attention. The reasons for this are threefold, and all have a major impact in the ideal of a 'profession' and any leadership strategy to take that ideal forward. A leader, to function well for a large population, must be visible. The role of the Chief Nursing Officer (CNO) has been central to that and in the past in England, as in the other UK countries, was supported in that role by a cadre of senior nurses drawn from most specialities. Their role was to advise the CNO and ministers on all aspects of nursing and midwifery, strongly promoting the role of these professions and their impact on quality care. The CNO role has more recently moved from one of accepted head of the profession to a barely visible figurehead supported in the main by secondees (temporary staff loaned to government by their employing organizations) who are unlikely to have vital organizational knowledge or to have had time to develop a powerbase to make much impact on professional issues. As well as the diminution of the CNO role, we have seen, in the UK, the demise of regional offices and the loss of the highly pivotal regional nurse director posts which had provided an important focus for development and succession planning across the regions and nationally. The more recently formed Special Health Authorities provide services to the whole of England. They are independent organizations with their own boards that include directors of nursing, but still fall under ministerial direction. Time will tell as to whether these nurses will achieve cohesive leadership. The opportunity exists for collegiate working and peer support through the Nurse Directors Association (NDA). This is an independent organization, with membership open to all nurse directors and senior nurses working in NHS organizations, and equivalent posts in the armed forces, independent sector, voluntary and charitable organizations in the UK. Given that historically, nurse leaders have risen in the main through the ranks of regions, this organization may go some way to meet the need for peer support, but its members are placed in a somewhat competitive position being employed by different health care trusts rather than by the government. This, combined with the gradual integration of senior nurses at trust level into the management framework, has eroded the opportunity for professional peer review, collegiate support and – most importantly – a degree of professional consensus at national level. This adds up to a profession in the UK that is successfully being marginalized from the leadership agenda at almost every level, despite making some very laudable advances in nurse-led initiatives at the clinical level.

Does this matter? Frustration at the nursing profession's apparent desire to be all things to all people and the concomitant manipulations by management to tread the paths of others may not be justified (Bishop 2002, 2004). If individuals can carve out for themselves careers which satisfy them, if quality control is handed to various agencies, and if nursing as a profession disappears into the integrated woodwork while generic health care workers pick up the hands-on aspects of health care, perhaps nursing as it has been identified over the past century is no longer needed. In which case one does wonder why a great deal of government and personal funding goes into degree courses for nursing. It is important to note here the massive impact that nursing has made on higher education, not only bringing in huge capital to universities for teaching commitments, but also creating an academic career structure which is only sometimes matched by essential resources in which the incumbents may flourish.

It seems that the nursing profession is at a very important point in its development and one which requires careful consideration if it is not just to survive but also to grow (Bishop and Freshwater 2004b: 196). Health care of today and into the future has the same complexity whether it is in developed or developing countries. The UK NHS has long been considered something of an ideal, and because of its size, leadership within its structures has become a critical issue. It is the largest European employer (NHS 2007) and the third largest world industry after the Red Army of China and the Indian Railway (NHS 2005). Never has clear leadership been more important if the NHS is to meet the demands of society, and never has nursing been in such a powerful position to improve the experience of patients. Maben and Griffiths (2008) rightly state that leadership and ownership are fundamental to the delivery of high quality care, and note that leadership has been one of the neglected elements of the UK reforms of recent years, echoing earlier words of Keyzer (1992), who considered that the nursing profession will have to adjust its strategies to suit the prevailing social climate. It could be argued that nursing has been too malleable and over-adjusted! Keyzer also argued that nurses will have to identify new leaders, adding that the choice is simple: the survival and growth of nursing, or its demise.

Conclusion

We have considered the components of leadership. There are views supporting *genetic, circumstantial and learned leadership origins*. Leadership cannot function effectively in a large organization without a power base, and that will derive from an *informational, authoritarian or charismatic base* – none of these being mutually exclusive. Through the case studies we can identify the ways in which effective leadership has been wielded, for good or ill, and the qualities and skills to be learned or honed for potential leaders.

We have also examined the structure, or lack of it, to support leadership in nursing and the allied professions in the UK. What is not highlighted in the above text is how to lead the largest professional workforce in the NHS, or any similar organization across the globe, nor how to determine shared values and beliefs globally. If there was an easy answer it would have been done! However, the following chapters address the complexities and offer some solutions. This chapter has identified the issues. Do we have a shared vision? I suspect not. Too many individual aims and too little professional cohesion. Nursing is slow to use the media, as if we are ashamed to come out from the shadows. Today the media can make or break individuals and organizations. The good or bad of this is not an issue for this text, but the importance of visibility is, and that visibility should not be tied to the government of the day but to the nursing profession and its ideals.

We have considered the power bases of leadership in theory, and how government policies over the past decades have tended to impact on nursing as a finite profession with a strong clinical focus. Multi- or interdisciplinary working can sometimes translate as 'de-professionalization'. Professional boundaries formally blurred in the UK with the introduction of reduced working hours for junior doctors, with nurses picking up some medical tasks (Department of Health (DoH) 1993). In the community, and in some specialized units, this blurring has long been informally practised, with a tacit understanding between the health care team, to the advantage of patients and staff. This in itself is no bad thing; however, *the power base for a profession must lie in the evidence of its effectiveness.* Despite the fact that most health care is delivered by teams, of which nurses are an essential part (Bloor and Maynard 1998, Maynard 1999 notes that most of the evidence base is dominated by doctors. This is a real chicken and egg situation – how do you get the egg without the chicken? Unless health care professionals are very clear as to their role and contribution to health care services, they will have difficulties in developing a power base of any significance. All professions that provide health care need to underpin that care with research and all employing organizations need to demonstrate that they are supporting staff in their professional development, and that they are good investors in people (Bishop and Freshwater 2004a).

It is in local areas that good leadership can be nurtured and honed, but would-be leaders must have good connections with the bigger picture and this means stepping out of the 'comfy zone' and mixing with peers from across the region, the country, and the wider profession across the world. Technology makes this possible. It also means being visible, articulate and with that wonderful energy of a passion and a vision to be shared. Leadership is not necessarily about destroying the status quo, although it may be. It can also be about strengthening it, and it is not reasonable to expect one person to meet all the leadership needs of a profession, or of a functioning group. Leaders are needed at every level in a large organization, and examples are highlighted in Chapters 4 and 5 of leadership initiatives that individuals have taken forward very successfully. Some of the leaders were heading a team, others had lead roles in a particular area and developed the services further, others led in a highly individual way, but they all stand out as leaders within their sphere. Perhaps what they all have in common is the courage to 'be a tall poppy' and stand above the rest. This does not necessarily make for comfortable living, as others may resent the attention given to these people. For those professionals who want to impact on a larger scale there are also unjust local preferences that may have to be managed when it comes to promotion. For example in the UK there was a period in the 1970s and 1980s when the fact that 90 per cent of the top nursing posts were held by men was widely cited. Today, despite the increase in black and minority ethnic health care staff in the NHS and the private sector, the percentage of executive posts held by them is still low. This is not a dilemma restricted to the UK; when a professorial post in nursing was created in Hong Kong over a decade ago (at time of writing) it was made quite clear to all interested parties that the incumbent had to be of Chinese origin. Such issues are not to be ignored, and undoubtedly cause some heartache. However, they are not a reason to give up! Policies are constantly changing, the world is shrinking with speedy travel and almost instant communication techniques, making old prejudices more and more irrelevant. This book will prepare any health care professional to lead in his or her field, if they want to.

Key points

- Leadership is essential to the effective functioning of groups and societies.
- Effective leadership involves having a vision, and the passion and intellect to sell it to your peers.
- A leader must have followers; this entails having good communications skills.
- Leadership ability may be inherited but it can certainly be learned.
- Leadership, to be successful, must have a power base, e.g. knowledge, funding, authority.
- Leadership may be transient, arising from changing circumstances.

Reflective exercises

1   Are there similarities between the leaders in the case studies? Does one kind of leadership style predominate in the group?
2   If you can imagine all six alive at the same time, and in the same environment, who do you think would be the leader? (*This may seem a silly question, but in considering a serious answer you will clarify many of the fundamental issues about leadership theory.*)
3   Consider the organization in which you work, and identify the leadership style that predominates there.
4   Write on one side of a page the attributes that you would like in a leader. On the other side, list how many of those that you consider that you have.
5   What formal opportunities exist where you work to network with colleagues? What external networks do you connect with?

6   The role of a follower is important, no leader can function without them. Do you connect with your current leader? Consider what skills you demonstrate to them.

7   List on one side of a page what special attributes you think that you would bring to a leadership role. On the other side, list what you think would be your weakest aspects as a leader. Then consider how you can improve on that.

References

Antrobus, S. (2003) What is political leadership? *Nursing Standard* 17(43): 40–44.

Bennis, W. (1997) *On Becoming a Leader*. London: Arrow.

Bennis, W. (1998) *Managing People is Like Herding Cats*. London: Kogan Page.

Bishop, V. (2002) Editorial. *Journal of Research in Nursing* 7(4): 240.

Bishop, V. (2004) Editorial. *Journal of Research in Nursing* 9(1): 4.

Bishop, V. and Freshwater, D. (2004a) Developing a research portfolio: building a professional profile. In D. Freshwater and V. Bishop (eds) *Nursing Research in Context: Appreciation, Application and Professional Development*. Basingstoke: Palgrave Macmillan.

Bishop, V. and Freshwater, D. (2004b) Looking ahead: the future for nursing research. In D. Freshwater and V. Bishop (eds) *Nursing Research in Context: Appreciation, Application and Professional Development*. Basingstoke: Palgrave Macmillan.

Bloor, K. and Maynard, A. (1998) Rewarding health care teams: a way of aligning pay to performance and outcomes. *British Medical Journal* 316(7131): 569.

Bottery, M. (1998) *Professionals and Policy: Management Strategy in a Competitive World*. London: Cassell.

Buchan, J. (2002) Editorials. Global nursing shortages. *British Medical Journal* 324: 751–752.

Buchan, J. (2004) Challenges of recruiting and retaining nurses: some thoughts for policy makers. *Journal of Research in Nursing* 8(4): 291–292.

Department of Health (DoH) (1993) *Hospital doctors: training for the future. Report of the Working Group on Specialist Medical Training* (Calman Report). London: DoH.

Department of Health and Social Security (DHSS) (1983) *NHS Management Enquiry* (Griffiths Report). London: DHSS.

Frank, M.S. (1993) The essence of leadership. *Public Personnel Management* 22(3); 381–389.

Galton, F. (1870). *Hereditary Genius*. New York: Appleton.

Gardner, J. (1989) *On Leadership*. New York: Free Press.

Girvin, J. (1998) *Leadership and Nursing*. Basingstoke: Palgrave Macmillan.

Greer, S. L. (2004) *Territorial Politics and Health Policy: The United Kingdom in Comparative Perspective*. Manchester: Manchester University Press.

Hennessy, D. (2000) The emerging themes. In D. Hennessy and P. Spurgeon (eds) *Health Policy and Nursing: Influence, Development and Impact*. London: Macmillan.

International Council of Nurses (ICN) (2001) *Leadership Bulletin: Leadership for Change Programme (LFC)*. Geneva: ICN.

Keyzer, D. (1992) Nursing policy, the supply and demand for nurses: towards a clinical career structure for nurses. In J. Robinson, A. Gray and R. Elkan (eds) *Policy Issues in Nursing*. Buckingham: Open University Press.

Lewin, K., Lippitt, R. and White, R.K. (1939) Patterns of aggressive behavior in experimentally created social climates. *Journal of Social Psychology* 10: 271–279.

Maben, J. and Griffith, P. (2008) *Nurses in Society: Starting the Debate*. London: King's College London.

Machiavelli, N. (1532) *Il Principe*, translated by P. Bondanella and M. Musa (1984) *The Prince*. Oxford: Oxford University Press.

Maslin-Prothero, S. and Masterson. A. (2002) Power, politics and nursing in the United Kingdom. *Policy, Politics, and Nursing Practice*. 3(2): 108–117.

Maynard, A. (1999) Clinical governance: commentary. The unavoidable economic challenges. *Nursing Times Research* 4(3): 189.

Mullins, L.J. (1999) *Management and Organisational Behaviour*, 5th edn. London: Financial Times Pitman.

Murray, S.J., Holmes, D. and Rail, G. (2008) On the constitution and status of 'evidence' in the health sciences. *Journal of Research in Nursing* 13(4): 272–280.

NHS (2005) Press release, 22 March.

NHS (2007) *NHS Careers*: www.nhscareers.nhs.uk.

Osseo-Asare, A.E., Longbottom, D. and Murphy, W.D. (2005) Leadership best practices for sustaining quality in UK higher education from the perspective of the EFQM Excellence Model. *Quality Assurance in Education*. 13(2): 148–170.

Roberts, A. (2004) *Hitler and Churchill: Secrets of Leadership*. London: Weidenfeld and Nicolson.

Robinson, J. (1992) Introduction: beginning the study of nursing policy. In J. Robinson, A. Gray and R. Elkan (eds) *Policy Issues in Nursing*. Buckingham: Open University Press.

Smith, P. and Peterson, M. (1988) *Leadership, Organisations and Culture*. London: Sage.

Stevens, J. (1997) Improving integration between research and practice as a means of developing evidence-based health care. *Nursing Times Research* 2(1): 7–15.

Stogdill, R. M. (1974) *Handbook of Leadership: A Survey of Theory and Research*. New York: Free Press.

Taffinder, P. (1995) *The New Leaders: Achieving Corporate Transformation through Dynamic Leadership*. London: Kogan Page.

Twinn, S. (2008) Professor of Nursing, Nethersole School of Nursing, The Chinese University of Hong Kong, personal communication.

Weber, M. (1947) *The Theory of Economic and Social Organisation*, translated by A.M. Henderson and T. Parson. New York: Free Press.

West, E. and Scott, C. (2000) Nursing in the public sphere: breaking the boundaries between research and policy. *Journal of Advanced Nursing* 32(4): 817–824.

Wilmot, S. (2003) *Ethics, Power and Policy: The Future of Nursing in the NHS*. Basingstoke: Palgrave.

Zairi, M. (1994) Leadership in TQM implementation: some case examples. *The TQM Magazine*, 6(6): 9–16.

2 Leadership and management: a new mutiny?

David Stanley

Overview

Are leadership and management different? In this chapter we explore this question, using the story of Bligh's expedition on HMS *Bounty* to illustrate key points. We will consider if role ambiguity exists for health professionals who hold clinical roles, but have management functions. Literature and research-based evidence suggest that conflict exists when clinicians assume management roles without appropriate training, support or instruction. The chapter concludes by proposing ways to deal with this dichotomy and provides evidence to support a more effective approach to management and leadership in the clinical domain.

Introduction

In this chapter we discuss the differences between leadership and management. The examples that I have studied involve nurses in the UK and in Australia, but the principles involved pertain to all professions allied to medicine. It is proposed that managers are mainly driven by their desire to maintain stability, control and administer people and resources, while clinical leaders are commonly identified and followed because they are approachable, open and clinically competent. They are seen as empowered decision makers, visible in the clinical area, effective communicators and positive clinical role models. This suggests that operating both a management and leadership function within the same post or person may be counterproductive and inefficient.

It should come as no surprise to most clinical staff that the best and most experienced clinical member of a ward or unit team is not necessarily going to make the most effective or successful manager. However, in terms of ward, unit or department management, employers appear to persist with the appointment of senior clinical staff into management posts, or worse, encourage clinical staff into management posts and then burden them further by asking them to retain clinical responsibilities. Employers may hope that by holding on to a small part of their original occupational role this will offset any discomfort caused by having to adapt to new or alien roles of management and control (some modern matrons and nurse consultants are in these positions, but so too are many ward managers and senior ward sisters). There has been a proliferation of 'leadership' training or courses to support the managerial development of clinical staff into management positions, but this too offers a flawed solution because if leadership and management are different, then what is required are courses that support the specific roles undertaken; that is leadership courses that address genuine leadership issues and management courses for people whose focus is on management. Until there is an acceptance that these functions are different, courses will continue to neglect to address the participants' specific requirements. The drive in the UK to have more clinicians in key leadership roles (Department of Health (DoH) 1999, 2000), while ideal, is hampered by a perpetual misunderstanding about the difference between leadership and management. The result of refusing to recognize and thus address this dichotomy has been conflict, confusion, a challenge to the clinician's values and beliefs, disassociation from the clinician's core clinical values, ineffective leadership and management and potentially dysfunctional clinical areas, all of which is detrimental to quality care (Stanley 2006a, 2006b).

In this chapter three pillars in support of these statements are presented, and a solution offered. First, we consider some of the literature that discusses evidence of conflict that exists when clinicians assume management roles. Second, we move on to consider much of the literature that outlines the differences between management and leadership. Third, evidence is provided from a research study where one of the key areas of investigation related to issues that effect clinical leadership and ward management (Stanley 2000). From this it is suggested that if clinicians are able to recognize the differences between leadership and management, nurses and the professions allied to medicine can support a more appropriate approach to clinical area management and the clinical care of patients and clients.

Role ambiguity

The Voyage of the *Bounty*: Part 1

On 23 December 1787 (a 'bleak, boisterous, cloudy day': Alexander 2003: 78) Lieutenant William Bligh set sail with a crew of 45 on a mission to collect Artocarpus Incisa (Breadfruit) from the island of Tahiti and transport it to the West Indies. The little cutter, *Bounty* was specifically fitted out for the task and Bligh was considered a good choice as commander. His role on the *Bounty*, was to ensure the ship was sailed skilfully, that appropriate sailors undertook specific functions throughout the journey, to oversee the health and welfare of the crew, including their food and rum supply, to set the course and to control discipline. On the *Bounty* he was lord and master and although he was denied use of the Master's cabin (this had been converted for the storage of Breadfruit) he was in sole charge of the mission. The King's Regulations and the Admiralty's instructions were Bligh's authority and standards and he was in sole control of the ship. However, was Bligh a leader or a manager?

Abraham Lincoln said, in 1858, 'A house divided against itself cannot stand.' He was referring to the nation of America, or at least the American Congress, where many of the states approved of slavery and many did not. I believe this is also true when applied to clinical staff whose focus is divided between clinical and professional values, and their management role and its associated responsibilities. Bishop refers in Chapter 1 to the disillusionment of many staff when the values of their employing organization are at odds with their core professional values and beliefs. Naughton and Nolan (1998) anticipated this when considering nursing's future role, indicating that the drive to offer more (managerial) power to nurses could create a number of tensions, especially between professional aspirations and the demands of a new managerial culture. They felt that 'many nurses have found themselves torn between the push towards the ideal of individualised holistic care and the reality of resource constrained environments (Naughton and Nolan 1998: 983). Forbes (1993) posited that traditional management tasks (i.e. staffing, staff evaluation, budgeting etc.) were best left to administrators because these duties would just cloud the clinical focus of senior clinical nurses; a conclusion supported by Doyal (1998: 9) who found that nurses appointed to managerial roles suffered from 'confusion of identity' that often led to 'anxiety and isolation for the post holders'. Doyal also indicated that ward managers and senior sisters 'felt uncertain about where to locate themselves, particularly in areas of professional identity, relations with colleagues and managerial responsibilities'.

More recently Firth (2002) further supported these findings following interviews with a sample of ward managers. 'Role ambiguity' was identified as a main theme and participants were found to be unclear about their role, even angry about how the role had evolved. The majority of managers interviewed indicated that if they could delegate the administrative side of their role to someone else their role would be improved, causing Firth to conclude that ward managers experience conflict between the management and clinical dimensions of their role. These findings are not new and certainly concur with my findings (Stanley 2000) when exploring the role of ward sisters in general ward areas. One participant in this study, when asked to discuss her role as a ward sister replied:

> "I think it is a role that is diminishing slightly. Ward sister, ward leader, ward manager, team leader, there are 101 names for it and I don't think it is respected very much in the NHS because it is a very difficult role straddling clinical and management. You never know quite where your boundaries are."

The study concluded that ward sisters struggled with limited support, limited resources and staff shortages. Participants were commonly ill-prepared for their role particularly in relation to leadership and quality issues, and increasingly expressed feelings of conflict in their work. This was due to their preconceived, traditional idea of what their role and responsibilities should be, set against the realities of a changing health service (Stanley 2000). These changes, or blurring of professional boundaries, were noted by Reed and Kent (1997) who attributed this to a loss of clear nursing leadership. Murphy et al. (1997: 34) also considered that there was confusion and vagueness about the role and function of ward managers 'characterised by complexity, loss of focus and role overlap'. Further evidence of this role conflict is offered by Willmot (1998), whose evaluation of the changing role of the charge nurse indicated that 72 per cent of charge nurses felt unable to find a balance between the two roles, while a similar number also expressed feelings of isolation from their peers and teams.

Added to these are the views derived from a study by Christian and Norman (1998) that explored the role of clinical leaders/managers in 28 Nursing Development Units in the UK. These units, funded from central government monies and managed by the King's Fund Centre, London, were set up to promote a more advanced approach to nursing practices, and indeed were the forerunners to subsequent formalization of advanced and specialist practice roles. What emerged from their investigation was that clinical leaders and managers were divided into two camps, with their ability to deploy leadership strategies being constrained in one way or another by their position in the organizational hierarchy. Those without strong managerial responsibilities had the capacity to develop a vision of the future, but had no authority to make that vision a reality. Those with day-to-day managerial responsibilities experienced difficulty in extracting themselves from the administrative issues so that they could think in strategic terms. The solution employed in the Nursing Development Units was to have the clinical leaders and managers achieve 'operational effectiveness' by supporting them to exercise authority and further managerial responsibility. However, findings from the study brought the authors to the conclusion that the 'solution ignored the important point that leadership and management may be very different and even conflicting activities and may not be easily combined in the same role' (Christian and Norman 1998: 114).

Malcolm et al. (2003: 654) also support the notion of a gap between the clinical culture and a governance or managerial culture, suggesting that clinical leaders should remain focused on professional issues, quality and care and not 'cross over to the other side' (i.e. management). In the UK, nurse consultants have been developed to occupy a clinical, quality and care development role. However, when Guest et al. (2001) investigated the nurse consultant role, they found that as well as being able to identify many positive areas within their work, nurse consultants also encountered problems. The authors identified these as role ambiguity, role overload, role conflict, role over lap and role boundary management issues.

These views support the earlier criticisms of Rowden (1998), who suggested that any nursing strategy needs to think more critically about the training needs of the clinical ward sisters (registered nurses). While it could be argued that considerable UK government investment in training through the NHS Modernization Agency and the NHS Leadership Centre has had some impact, a focus on skills related to leadership and management may not address the core issue affecting frontline registered nurses, sisters, ward managers, charge nurses, modern matrons or nurse consultants, who commonly feel conflict from having to balance the managerial and clinical demands of their post (Forbes 1993; Doyal 1998; Stanley 2000, 2006a, 2006b; Firth 2002). The regularity with which the issue of role conflict and blurred role boundaries appears in the literature points perhaps to a fault in the structure of ward/unit management. Clearly the perception that many nurses have, that the best clinical nurse may not be the best ward/unit manager, rings true and needs further consideration. If there is role conflict, confusion and a disassociation from the clinician and their core clinical values, could it be because leadership and management are two different things?

Leadership and management: different?

From my perspective it's unequivocal, the answer is 'Yes!' Some people will argue that the answer is 'No', because some managers can lead or because some leaders manage. However, there is much more to both leadership and management than a title. For example, I would argue that while I am very good at heating a pizza in an oven, I would hardly consider myself a chef, but I will return to the story of the Bounty to take this point further.

The Voyage of the *Bounty*: Part 2

The voyage of the *Bounty* was largely uneventful. The original plan had been to round Cape Horn and so approach Tahiti from the east. However, bad weather forced the *Bounty* back across the Atlantic Ocean and on around the Cape of Good Hope, across the Indian Ocean, south of New Holland, Van Diemen's Land and New Zealand and on to Tahiti across the South Pacific Ocean. Once in Tahiti there was a delay. The longer than anticipated voyage had meant they had arrived too late to harvest the Breadfruit so the crew and Bligh had to wait months for the plants to be in a transportable state. To this point Bligh had managed things very well. The journey was safe, discipline was appropriate (not as some have suggested, excessive), the crew had reasonable liberty and by all accounts enjoyed the many pleasures offered in Tahiti.

The reasons for the mutiny that occurred on the *Bounty* shortly after leaving Tahiti, fully loaded with Breadfruit, are still open to interpretation. There had been a number of incidents where Bligh had reason to question and admonish his officers and crew in the long wait for the Breadfruit to mature and there was some suggestion that men had become attached to the favours of some of the Tahitian women. Whatever the reasons, Bligh and 18 members of his crew were cast adrift in a 23-foot launch. Fletcher Christian was left with the remainder of the crew and the *Bounty* sailed into infamy.

It was at this point, off the island of Tofua, 3618 miles from the closest known area of civilization that Bligh was to demonstrate his leadership capabilities. Up until the point of the mutiny Bligh had been in control (or so he thought). He had done his best to maintain stability, keep the status quo. He had been involved with planning, resources management, goal setting and targets, organizing and staffing, controlling, problem solving and coping with the complexity of their mission. But the mutiny had brought about a change and Bligh could have buckled under the insult, humiliation and stress. But he didn't. He describes himself feeling 'an inward happiness' (Alexander 2003: 143) and he took to the task of getting this little boat and his meagre crew back to England. It was at this point that Bligh had to be a leader, realigning his crew to their new circumstance, setting direction and navigating, motivating and inspiring the dispirited crew, establishing his credibility as a commander and navigator and selling his vision for how they were to survive. All the time anticipating change and finding ways to cope with it.

Zaleznik (1977: 61) suggests that, 'managers and leaders are two very different types of people'. He adds that the conditions favourable to the growth of one may even be detrimental to the other. In his view managers and leaders have different attitudes towards their goals, careers, relations with others and themselves. He considers that managers' goals arise out of necessity rather than desires, that managers excel at diffusing conflict between individuals or departments, placating all sides while ensuring that an organization's day-to-day business gets done. His view of leaders, on the other hand, is that their goals arise from a personal or passionate desire to infuse meaning into the world. Leaders, he maintains, are about people and meaning, while managers like to work with people, they tend to maintain a low level of 'emotional' involvement and may withdraw from the meaning of events. Managers, he indicates, are seen as fairly passive people, intent on keeping the show on the road. However, leaders seem to be more solitary, proactive, intuitive, emphatic and attracted to situations of high risk. Leaders ask the 'why not' question and 'do the right thing', while managers 'do things right' (Bennis and Nanus 1985).

Strongly supporting these views are those posited by Kotter (1990) who also considers leadership and management to be two different things, each having their own function and their own characteristic activities. In his view management is about controlling and putting appropriate structures and systems in place. He describes managers as being involved with planning and budgeting, setting goals and targets, organizing and staffing, problem solving and coping with complexity.

Management is indeed co-dependent upon complexity, and modern management has evolved because without good management large organizations and complex enterprises tended to become chaotic. Good managers bring order and consistency to key dimensions like quality and profitability.

The Voyage of the *Bounty*: Part 3

The boat had a shallow beam and they threw overboard all excess items, they had limited food and water and were attacked when they tried to land on Tofua to replenish their stores (one of the crew was killed). The launch took 48 days to reach Coupang on the Island of Timor. Bligh achieved this with no charts and while he had a compass, his sextant was broken and unreliable. They had to endure starvation rations and suffered from hunger, thirst and exposure as well as the constant danger of being in a small boat on a large and dangerous ocean in a strange and hostile part of the world. However, under Bligh's leadership they all arrived safely in the Dutch East Indies. Sadly some of the crew were now so weak that they were to die shortly after their deliverance, though most survived to return to England with Bligh nine months later.

Leadership differs. It is about coping with change, responding to chaos or creating chaos to some extent. Part of the reason it has become such an issue, particularly in relation to current health service needs, is that more change always demands more leadership (Kotter 1990) and few people could argue that change hasn't been a constant feature of the recent health care landscape. However, leadership has more to do with aligning people, setting direction, motivating, inspiring, employing credibility, adopting a visionary position, anticipating change and coping with change. While acknowledging that both management and leadership are necessary for the functioning of complex organizations, Kotter (1990) emphasizes their differences. Leadership seems to be rooted in the maxim that the more change there is, the more leadership is required. While supportive of Kotter's views, Warren (2005) is more specific, indicating that 'vision' is the main difference between leadership and management. Management, he states, consists primarily of three things:

- Analysis
- Problem solving
- Planning.

Warren (2005) considers that a leader is essentially able to clarify the purpose of an activity, stating that leadership consists of:

- Vision
- Values
- Communication of these things.

From this perspective, leaders could be described as the 'heart of an organization', with the essence of leadership being to inspire a group to come together for a common goal. Leaders motivate, console and work with people to keep them bonded and eager to move forward. This means setting direction, communicating it to everyone and keeping people on track when times get tough. Bligh's journey on the launch is a good example of this description of leadership.

Transformational and transactional: different?

Although the distinctions between different types of leadership are well described by Bishop in Chapter 1, it is useful here to revisit the differences between transformational and transactional styles in order to cut through the web of confusion between leadership and management. Transformational leadership (Downton 1973; Burns 1978) is strongly associated with

Bass (1985, 1990) and his work to try and tease out the distinctions between management associated with 'transactional leadership', and leadership associated with 'transformational leadership'. Transformational leadership is described as a process that changes and transforms individuals (Northouse 2004). It involves emotions, motives, ethics, long-term goals and an exceptional form of influence that moves the followers to accomplish more than is usually expected of them, incorporating both charismatic and visionary leadership (Northouse 2004). Kenneth Leithwood (1999, cited in Day et al. 2000) in considering transformational leadership from an educational perspective indicated that it involves setting directions, establishing a vision, developing people, organizing and building relationships.

Transactional leadership (Burns 1978), however, is based on the exchange relationship between the leader and the followers. The role of a transactional leader is to focus upon the purposes of the organization and to assist people to recognize what needs to be done in order to reach a desired outcome (Day et al. 2000). Also known as 'transactional management', transactional leadership is associated with the skill and ability to deal with the mundane, operational and day-to-day transactions of organizational life (Kakabadse and Kakabadse 1999).

Management and leadership: mind and spirit

Managers can be described as the brains of a business or organization. They establish systems, create rules and operating procedures and they put into place incentive programmes and the like. *Management however, is about the business, not about the people.* The people, therefore, are important only as a way of getting the job done. Managers have subordinates and they emphasize rationality and control focused on goals, resources, organizational structures or people management. While leaders have followers, are imaginative, passionate, non-conforming, risk takers, and work from the perspective of their vision or values. The case studies in Chapter 1 highlight this, believing in a 'universal truth' with which to rally their followers.

For some time, concepts and descriptions of management and leadership have been used interchangeably. Field (2002), however, describes leadership as being about taking action and communicating values in context of a relationship. It is *not* about reinforcing the status quo and reliance on hierarchy. As such, Field suggests that it is time to lay to rest the false confusion about leadership definitions and accept that leadership is different from management, that leadership applies to all kinds of people at all levels in organizations and that leadership is about relationships. Field Marshal Sir William Slim said of managers that they are necessary, but leaders are essential. Leadership is of the spirit, compounded of personality and vision; management is of the mind, more a matter of accurate calculation, statistics, methods, timetables and routine.

Management and leadership can therefore be described as two different concepts (see Table 2.1). Management is a function that must be exercised in any business or organization. Leadership is a relationship between the leader and the led that can energize an organization or business. But they are different things. Bennis and Nanus (1985), famous for their study of leadership and management, describe a leader as someone who is able to develop and communicate a vision which gives meaning to the work of others, but they add that most organizations are managed – not lead.

To come back to our example of Captain Bligh's journey, his management of the *Bounty* was an example of accurate calculation, established methods, timetables, control, duty and discipline. He was reasonably effective in this regard, but only to a point. For somewhere in the Pacific Ocean, Bligh lost control and Fletcher Christian was able to lead a small group of the crew in a successful mutiny. Fletcher Christian was a leader with passion, personal charisma and a determined group of followers. He acted proactively, sold his ideas successfully, broke the rules and managed to set a new direction by linking or latching onto the values and aspirations of a select few and leading them to liberate the *Bounty* from Bligh.

The Voyage of the *Bounty*: Part 4

Most of the crew didn't mutiny. Most driven by duty or fear or out of loyalty stayed with Bligh. Some of the crew were pressed into staying with the mutineers, to help sail the *Bounty* or because their skills were considered essential. But it was after the mutiny that Bligh showed that he too could be a leader. He led with passion (for his crew's survival and his personal hope of revenge or vindication), sold his ideas for survival, broke the rules, helped set a new direction by being flexible in the face of constant changes in their situation and because he was also linked to the values and hopes of the crew. His management skills were also essential, for he managed their scarce resources with great skill. But it was his leadership ability, not his management talents, that brought them all safely back to civilization.

Table 2.1   Summary view of the differences between leadership and management

AREA/FACTOR	LEADERSHIP	MANAGEMENT
Aims	Change	Stability/status quo
Objectives	Communication of vision Expression of values	Achievement of organizational aims or objectives
Theoretical approach	Transformational or congruent	Transactional
Relationship with conflict	Uses conflict constructively	Avoids or manages conflict
Relationship to power	Personal charisma/ personality/values	Formal authority/ hierarchical position
Blame/responsibility	Takes the blame	Tends to blames others/ processes
Core energy	Passion	Control
Relationship to the led/managed	Followers	Subordinates
Creativity	Explores new roads	Travels on existing paths
Main focus	Leading people	Managing work/tasks/ people
Planning	Sets direction	Plans detail
Motivation from	Heart/spirit	Head/mind
Response pattern	Proactive	Reactive
Persuasion style	Sell	Tell
Personal motivation	Excitement for work/ unification of values	Money or other tangible reward/getting job done
Relationship to rules	Breaks or explores the boundary of rules	Makes or keeps rules
Approach to risk	Takes risks	Minimizes risk
Approach to the future	Creates new opportunities	Establish systems/ processes
Who within an organization	Anyone/everyone	Those with specific senior hierarchical positions
Relationship to the organization	Essential	Necessary

New research perspectives

Research on clinical nurse leadership brought to light key themes that addressed participants' understanding of the differences between management and leadership (Stanley 2006b). The research involved three phases: a questionnaire (n=830), in-depth interviews with a random selection of nurses of different grades in four different clinical areas or units, and finally further interviews with nurses nominated as clinical leaders during the initial interviews. For the purposes of this chapter the focus is on the results of the interviews that questioned participants specifically about leadership, management and the difference between the two. They were also asked how this impacted on their role. The consensus drawn was that managers tended to depend on their position, title and hierarchical status, while leaders depended upon their ability to inspire people, relying instead on their knowledge and experience.

In general, managers were commonly seen as having 'more authority than a leader' and leadership was seen as 'not necessarily grade related ... it is a quality that some people have ... the ability to inspire colleagues'. Another participant said the difference was that 'the manager has got the title, and therefore they manage because of the title, but there are other people that lead by virtue of their opinion'.

Some participants emphasized the interpersonal relationship aspect of leadership describing leaders in terms of 'dealing with people, while management was more about dealing with systems and processes'. Supporting this perspective another participant indicated that:

"Leadership involves everybody ... leadership is more about guiding people, it's about talking to people, being on their wavelength, seeing how they feel, seeing what they are capable of doing. Management to me is more office based, managing the people that are working for you. Managing budgetary constraints and things like that."

Others said that 'management was about being controlled' , or that 'managers found it difficult to get properly involved'. Describing the difference between managing and clinical leadership, many offered views about the diminished clinical input of managers, one said:

"Managers are very good ... unfortunately for them they are no longer clinical. They do clinical shifts, but they are so bogged down with everything else that's going on with national initiatives such as NICE [the National Institute for Health and Clinical Excellence] and all the paperwork that's involved with it. I would say that on the shopfloor, as we used to say, that it was the sisters and staff nurses and there are some exceptional ones that are the leaders."

Another, describing her ward manager, said:

> "Sometimes perhaps she is not very approachable. You feel that you know she's obviously busy doing the managerial stuff and actual running the ward ... doing the day-to-day things rather than being able to support the staff clinically ... she doesn't carry much of a clinical workload, she is more administrative."

When asked if there were issues about being a leader or manager, one participant said that 'being a manager ... it was sometimes hard to either do one or the other', and another replied that 'management and leadership are totally separate entities ... there are barriers, especially the higher up the ladder you get, you get focused on the clerical side and the patient care can suffer'. A number of participants saw 'barriers between the two'. Indicating that they were so separate that, as one respondent said, 'I think you can perhaps get somebody that knows nothing about nursing and you can put them in a management position, you know they probably could do the job', a view echoed by another, 'they could pick someone off the street and make them into a decent manager, but leadership comes from within ... it's different'.

Supporting the notion of a division between the functions of leaders and managers, another participant said, 'I suppose a leader would be more involved with the actual work, whereas a manager would be more involved with the paperwork and that sort of thing'.

Other participants described managers as 'distant from the ward', 'more interested in the finance and things', 'more office based' , 'hidebound' or having 'more authority than a leader'.

In order to clarify who participants saw as a manager or leader, each participant was specifically asked if the modern matron or their ward manager was seen as a leader or manager. One participant said:

> "I don't see her [matron] as clinical and she is not somebody I would admire in the same way as a clinical nurse. Although she is obviously clinical she's lost a lot of the clinical skills purely because she does what she does and I think she is all tied up with administration and management and finances and that just comes out every time."

She then added:

> "I think when she was first appointed I did initially think why can't we have say ... another two or three D grade nurses instead of another tier of management. I just saw her as another stick to beat us with. I thought why can't we just employ more nurses to come and do the work."

Another describing her modern matron said:

"We've got a matron who is mainly office based ... managing staff, beds, finances, and things like that, whereas if you've got somebody who's based within the ward setting they're going to be more of a clinical leader."

This view of the modern matron was again repeated from another locality, 'they are basically ... you know 80% of the time they are sat in the office doing something ... it's like a supervisory role'. As one participant said, 'I think she is seen as a manager, she's simply not involved on the ward [clinical activity] every day.'

Clearly there was some dissonance between the intention of the UK Department of Health (2000: 86) that modern matrons were to be a 'strong clinical leader with clear authority at ward level' and the perspective of many of the participants in this study. This disparity is summed up in these comments where it is suggested that:

"Management could diminish your impact as a leader. The negative side of nursing promotion is the fact that there is a greater tendency to come off the shop floor which can tend to diminish your impact as a leader."

"Within nursing the emphasis for promotion seems to be put upon managerial skills and it has been certainly in the 20 years that I've been in and out of nursing that seems to be ... well ... I would love to see clinical excellence rewarded."

Recognizing that leaders were found at all levels and in a range of different areas, a number of participants described leaders as 'someone who doesn't have to be in a management position', 'someone inspirational', 'someone who comes with knowledge and experience'. Leadership and management were clearly seen as different things, although a relationship existed between them. Managers were seen as further removed from care, climbing the managerial career ladder, but at the same time sliding down the professional nurse snake in terms of clinical credibility, effectiveness or their capacity to lead clinically. Clinical leaders could come from any level, advancing clinical care because they were approachable, inspirational, visible, clinically skilled, experienced and most importantly driven by their core nursing and care values.

Interviews with those nurses who received the most nominations as clinical leaders identified two issues in relation to differences between management and leadership – 'juggling everything' and 'conflict'. A major preoccupation appeared to be with balancing their clinical and managerial responsibilities. For example, as one interviewee said:

"I see myself as having two priorities. One is the patients, obviously, that's what we're here for, and my second is my staff ... if there is a conflict between staff requirements and patient requirements, the patient requirements come first."

Others implied that they would be happier if they didn't have to deal with the management aspects of their role.

> "It would be wonderful ... without a doubt ... you know I mean I'd rather not be dealing with people's salaries ... annual leave request ... monitoring sickness ... because I would be far more valuable out on the ward working along side junior colleagues."

> "My role is patient care. I am accountable for everything I do for my patients. I would say that this is my major role."

> "I would like to have more influence to change things, but having said that I wouldn't particularly want to go down the management road and get involved with all the meetings and committees and all that sort of thing, but from a clinical perspective I'd like to have more influence."

Clinical leaders described themselves as being driven by their 'beliefs about patient care' and they spoke of their desire to apply *and* display high quality care. Conflict arose when management responsibilities were seen to diminish their effectiveness as clinical leaders. This was summed up neatly by one participant:

> "The more management responsibility you've got, the less you are visible in the clinical area. There is only so much you can do which is one of the reasons why I don't want to go any further [with my career]."

Not only were leadership and management different, but also the clinical leaders and the majority of the other nurses interviewed clearly indicated that taking on management responsibilities were likely to be detrimental to the fulfilment of a clinician's clinical leadership capacity.

Is there another way?

These findings support the not inconsiderable evidence quoted previously that management and leadership functions embodied in the same person, or within the same post lead to confusion, conflict and diminished clinical and management effectiveness. Addressing this issue must surely be considered central to improving the efficiency of clinical areas and to developing sustainable improvements in the quality of patient or client care. One solution is to divide the two roles and to create posts where either management or clinical leadership are the goals. An option could be the creation of administrators whose purpose would be to manage wards or units on a day-to-day basis, dealing with clerical duties, staffing issues, stores, stock, safety issues, risk assessments, complaints and the administrative duties essential for effective functioning. A post to support clinical staff, much like a pit crew support a racing driver, necessary, functional, but secondary to the main event. Experienced clinical staff could then be gifted with the freedom to lead clinical care, focusing on quality, and the provision of expert and experienced care to clients and patients. These are the staff who should be consulted by administrators before significant decisions affecting the ward or unit are made. Modern matrons, clinical nurses and ward sisters could retain a strong influence over the clinical direction and quality issues of the ward or unit. They could effectively support junior or neophyte colleagues, offer direct examples of high quality care, be visible and approachable role models, and leave behind the conflict and confusion about role boundaries prevalent in the current ward or unit structures.

Such a change in traditional structures within the UK somewhat turns the tables on Griffith's vision for management within the NHS (DHSS 1983), which were supposed to offer career opportunities for nurses but in fact helped to propagate the conflict and confusion described above. Bishop notes in Chapter 1 that Griffiths was not beneficial to nursing or to the provision of nursing care as it took nurses away from the bedside and helped to split the nursing workforce that had never truly been cohesive. A house divided cannot stand and it is time to recognize the divisions that the current approach to ward or unit or department management effects. The cultural shift to achieve this would be tremendous and has implications for the provision of appropriate continuing professional development and indeed a political shift in health care policy. However, the potential benefits in terms of improvements to patient care and staff retention could be tremendous too.

Case study 2.1 Horses for courses

A practical example of this approach is offered here. I was once the manager of a children's services department in the north of England. On the paediatric ward that I oversaw there was a nurse's aide who had injured her back, but wanted to return to work. She couldn't do so in a clinical capacity. There was also a senior ward sister who spent most of her day dealing with health and safety assessments, rosters, ordering stock and very, very little time doing what she loved doing and for what she had spent years learning – caring for sick and ill children. So my solution was to replace the senior nurse with the injured nurse's aide. She came to work for four hours each day and sorted ward stores and stocks, assessed health and safety issues and did the rosters. There was considerable opposition from some clinical staff. Qualified nurses didn't like a non-registered nurse doing their rosters (although she did a great job). Non-qualified nurses didn't like one of their colleagues becoming a 'manager' although we never used this term. The registered children's nurse, however, was delighted to be free of the management duties to focus again on the sick children. The injured nurse's aide was very happy to have four hours work each day that didn't aggravate her back and I was delighted that we now had one more highly experienced and skilled children's nurse caring for the children and a motivated and satisfied member of staff contributing to the ward. It should have been a win/win situation, but staff opposition (in spite of the obvious advantages), because it wasn't a traditional ward management model, meant that as soon as I left and moved on to another post the approach was curtailed and I gather the previous model was reinstituted. Sadly, this approach was never formally evaluated before it was discontinued and a genuinely positive opportunity to offer a new approach to ward adminis-tration was lost.

The case study serves to emphasize the differences between leadership and management, supporting the views of researchers in this field. The signifi-cance of these differences in relation to clinical care, and the management of clinical areas, is conflict, confusion and a possible division between core clinical values and organizational goals.

Different perspectives

Part of my aim in outlining this perspective is to challenge some long-held and unproductive views of how health care organizations function. While some managers consider these views to be unfair, they represent those of some very well published and scholarly people (Zaleznik 1977; Kotter 1990; Field 2002; Robbins 2002; Warren 2005). My point is that the health service is always in a state of flux and to cope with change, organizations need leaders and sometimes it *is* the manager who fulfils this role, while at other times others within the organization lead. To suggest that only managers can lead would be a mistake. Maintaining the status quo requires considerable energy; and working as a manager in the health service requires resilience, commitment and dedication and I am not having a go at managers. I am, however, making a case for others to be seen as leaders, which may shake the status quo and this could be seen as threatening. Managers are about stability, managing the organization and keeping things on an even keel. Some managers are able to lead and engage in both the stable management tasks and creative risk taking leadership – but this is rare. Maintaining the status quo is commonly vital and requires often huge amounts of energy applied in creative ways; managers are generally very good at this. But this isn't leadership and it isn't about change or about actions to make or take change.

Appointing and training people who are asked to function as managers, but with expectations that they will offer dynamic and risk taking leadership sets them up to fail or leads them to feel insecure in their role. These practices are almost epidemic in proportion. No one wins and health services suffer. Clinical leadership and management responsibilities are therefore placed in positions of diminished clinical effectiveness, or in a weakened managerial position (Christian and Norman 1998). Ward managers, senior sisters, nurse consultants, modern matrons and a whole host of other senior clinical staff with managerial responsibilities find themselves climbing the managerial ladder, only to slide down the clinical snake! Advancing themselves or their organization's objectives is too often at the cost of effective clinical leadership, often depriving neophyte nurses and unskilled or semi-trained carers at the bedside, of their guidance and clinical leadership that could really improve patient and client care.

For a genuine opportunity to develop more efficient ward or unit management and clearer, more effective clinical leadership it may be time to accept that having leadership and management functions reside in one person or post is inefficient and counterproductive, both to the individual concerned and the health service's future development and success.

Key points

- Leadership and management are different.
- Misunderstanding the differences can lead to conflict, confusion, a challenge to the clinician's values and beliefs, disassociation from the clinician's core clinical values, and ineffective leadership and management.
- There is considerable evidence that management and leadership functions, embodied in the same person or within the same post, lead to confusion, conflict and diminished clinical and management effectiveness.
- Nurse managers and a whole host of other senior clinical nurses with managerial responsibilities find themselves climbing the managerial ladder at the expense of their clinical career. Advancing themselves or the Trust's objectives at the cost of effective clinical leadership.
- There may be other, more effective, more productive and more satisfying models for the facilitation of management and leadership approaches in clinical areas.

Reflective exercises

1   Are leadership and management different? Speak with a registered nurse, ward manager (or whatever they are called in your clinical area) and see if they have a view about this.

2   Do nurses' job titles matter? Think about this. Why do we have the job titles we do? What does it mean to be a registered nurse, sister, a ward manager, a clinical nurse or a nurse consultant?

3   Take a sheet of paper. On the right-hand side make a list of the characteristics and qualities you would seek in a good or effective manager. On the left make a list the characteristics and qualities you would seek in a good or effective leader. Compare the lists. Are they the same? Where are they different?

4   Think about your nurse education. What did you learn about management? Was this adequate? Do you think there are other matters or topics that nurses should learn about to ensure they are skilled managers (e.g. financial management, human resources management)? Did your general nurse education prepare you or other nurses to function as effective managers?

5   What did you learn about leadership? Was this topic covered in your curriculum? Talk about this with nursing students or qualified colleagues. Has the nursing curriculum changed over the years to support better nurse management or leadership training?

References

Alexander, C. (2003) *The Bounty*. London: HarperCollins.

Bass, B.M. (1985) *Leadership and Performance Beyond Expectations*. New York: Free Press.

Bass, B.M. (1990) From transactional to transformational leadership: learning to share the vision. *Organisational Dynamics*. 18: 19–31.

Bennis, W. and Nanus, B. (1985) *Leaders: The Strategies for Taking Charge*. New York: Harper and Row.

Burns, J.M. (1978) *Leadership*. New York: Harper and Row.

Christian, S.L. and Norman, I.J. (1998) Clinical leadership in Nursing Development Units. *Journal of Advanced Nursing* 27: 108–116.

Day, C., Harris, A., Hadfield, M., Tolley, H. and Beresford, J. (2000) *Leading Schools in Times of Change*. Buckingham: Open University Press.

Department of Health (1999) *Making a Difference*. London: Stationery Office.

Department of Health (2000) *The NHS Plan*. London: Stationery Office.

Department of Health and Social Security (DHSS) (1983) *NHS Management Enquiry* (Griffiths Report). London: DHSS.

Downton, J.V. (1973) *Rebel Leadership: Commitment and Charisma in a Revolutionary Process*. New York: Free Press.

Doyal, L. (1998) Crossing professional boundaries. *Nursing Management* 5(4): 8–10.

Field, R.G.H. (2002) *Leadership Defined: Web Images Reveal the Difference between Leadership and Management*. Administrative Sciences Association of Canada 2002 Annual Meeting: www.busualberta.ca/rfield/papers/Leadershipdefined.htm

Firth, K. (2002) Ward leadership: balancing the clinical and managerial roles. *Professional Nurse* 17(8): 486–489.

Forbes, K. (1993) Management does not equal leadership. *Nursing Management* 7(3): 129.

Guest, D., Peccei, R., Rosenthal, P., Montgomery, J., Redfern, S., Young, C., Wilsons-Barnet, J., Dewe, P., Evans, A. and Oakley, P. (2001) *A Preliminary Evaluation of the Establishment of Nurse Midwife and Health Visitor Consultants.* London: Department of Health and King's College London.

Kakabadse, A. and Kakabadse, N. (1999) *Essence of Leadership.* London: International Thomson Business Press.

Kotter, J.P. (1990) *What Leaders Really Do.* Boston, MA: Harvard Business School Press.

Malcolm, L., Wright, L., Barnett, P. and Hendry, C. (2003) Building a successful partnership between management and clinical leadership: experience from New Zealand. *British Medical Journal* 326: 653–654.

Murphy, E.C., Ruch, S., Pepicello, J. and Murphy, M. (1997) Managing an increasingly complex system. *Nursing Management* 28(10): 33–38.

Naughton, M. and Nolan, M. (1998) Developing nursing's future role: a challenge for the millennium. *British Journal of Nursing* 7(16): 983–986.

Northouse, P.G. (2004) *Leadership: Theory and Practice*, 3rd edn. London: Sage.

Reed, L. and Kent, S. (1997) New nursing structures. *Nursing Management* 4(1): 18–20.

Robbins, S. (2002) The difference between managing and leading. *Entrepreneur.com* 18 November: www.entrepreneur.com/management/leadership/article 57304.html

Rowden, R. (1998) Unleashing the potential. *Nursing Times* 94(43): 62–63.

Stanley, D. (2000) In the trenches. Unpublished MSc thesis, Birmingham University, UK.

Stanley, D. (2006a) In command of care: towards the theory of congruent leadership. *Journal of Research in Nursing* 2(2): 134–144.

Stanley, D. (2006b) Recognising and defining clinical nurse leaders. *British Journal of Nursing* 15(2): 108–111.

Warren, R. (2005) What's the difference between managing and leading? *Transforming Churches*: http://transformingchurch.com/resources/2005/08whats_the _dif.php

Willmot, M. (1998) The new ward manager: an evaluation of the changing role of the charge nurse. *Journal of Advanced Nursing* 28: 419–427.

Zaleznik, A. (1977) Managers and leaders are they different? *Harvard Business Review: On Leadership* 61–88. Boston, MA: Harvard Business School Press.

3 Leadership challenges: professional power and dominance in heath care

Mike Saks

Overview

In this chapter we consider the leadership challenges posed by professional power and dominance in health care in the Anglo-American context. Outlining the nature of professions, including their legally defined power base and the way in which some have become particularly dominant, the classic example of the relationship between medicine and nursing and the allied health professions is highlighted. Traditionally, professions have been viewed positively as altruistic groups of experts committed to public protection. However, recently a more critical stance has been taken towards professional groups in which concerns have been raised about how they have used their power and dominance more in their own interests than those of the wider public, and again examples are drawn from health care. In conclusion, the implications for leadership in the health professions in dealing with the challenges of professional power and dominance are discussed.

Introduction

In this chapter we examine from an historical and contemporary viewpoint the leadership challenges posed by professional power and dominance in health care, which has longstanding roots in the Anglo-American context. As is discussed fully in Chapter 2, leadership in this sense is distinguished from management that involves performing specific functions in an organization related to formal positions co-ordinating or controlling organizational activities (Bratton et al. 2007). Members of professional bodies may hold such roles in organizations, but the leadership challenge discussed here is more about the influence such players or those who interact with them wield in encouraging positive behaviour towards clients and/or wider societal goals. This may be either through members of professions themselves pursuing positive objectives and visions of the future, or through stimulating members of professions to follow in this direction in terms of values and beliefs (Brooks 2006). As such, leadership may require both professions and professionals or those interacting with them to reinforce the status quo and/or act as change agents. First, we have to outline the nature of professions in order to understand their patterns of power and dominance in health care specifically.

The nature of the health care professions

The range of professions in modern society is now large, spanning from architecture and accountancy to law and medicine. In the northern hemisphere such groups can be seen as relatively distinctive to Britain and the United States, on which this chapter focuses. Despite variations in their history and form, the characteristic independence of such occupations in these two countries differentiates them from those in much of continental Europe. In continental Europe these occupational groups lie more on a spectrum in terms of autonomy towards the end of which lie state-centrist societies like France and the former Soviet Union, where groups such as doctors and nurses were subordinate to the party and the socialist state (Macdonald 1995). Those professions with greatest independence in the Anglo-American context tend to stand at the top of the occupational pecking order. There is little doubt that in this respect – in an era of biomedical ascendancy – medicine as a profession has for long been at the apex of the health care hierarchy in both Britain and the United States as compared to nursing and other allied health professions (Saks 2003a).

Having said this, such professions are formally considered here in terms of a neo-Weberian perspective which takes a politicized approach, seeing professions as particular types of occupational groups that have effected social closure through political action, and by creating legally defined boundaries that exclude outsiders. From this perspective, work structures are viewed as emerging from the relationships between occupations in health (and other areas), as they vie with each other on the basis of their competing group interests in the marketplace (Saks 2003b). Occupations that manage to gain their autonomy by winning the approval of the state are able to regulate market conditions in their favour by constructing legally enshrined divisions between privileged insiders and disenfranchised outsiders. Such 'professional' groups benefit through the associated increase in income, status and power that is achieved by socially excluding competitors. This process generates relationships of domination and subordination both among professions themselves and in relation to occupations that lie outside their boundaries – the precise nature of which depends on the form of professionalization involved. This is now highlighted with reference to the development of health care professions in the Anglo-American context, as a backcloth to the ensuing discussion about leadership challenges.

Perspectives from the UK

In Britain prior to the mid-nineteenth century there was a wide range of therapies on offer in a relatively pluralistic environment and no national system of legally sustained exclusionary closure in health care (Saks 2003a). However, the 1858 Medical Registration Act provided for a legally underwritten, self-regulating medical profession – which for the first time unified apothecaries, surgeons and physicians and created a medically dominated General Medical Council (GMC) with central responsibility for education and training, maintaining a professional register and overseeing internal disciplinary matters (Waddington 1984). Although this did not formally preclude outsiders from operating under the Common Law as long as they did not claim to be registered medical practitioners, it did create a de facto monopoly of practice and led to upward collective social mobility for the vast majority of doctors in terms of income, status and power (Parry and Parry 1976). Their position, moreover, was later reinforced through the 1911 National Health Insurance Act and the 1946 National Health Insurance Act that enabled the medical profession to monopolize the market in the fast-growing public sector. This was further supported by legislation in the first half of the twentieth century that restricted the conditions – such as cancer and diabetes – that the non-medically qualified could claim to treat in both the public and the private sector (Larkin 1995).

Thus the medical profession became the first and most powerful health profession in Britain. It went from strength to strength with the rise of 'scientific' biomedicine that developed from eighteenth-century 'bedside medicine', in which rich clients controlled diagnosis and treatment, to nineteenth- and twentieth-century 'hospital medicine' and 'laboratory medicine', in which the patient became disempowered and subordinated to the doctor (Jewson 1976). In tandem with the emergence of a medical elite drawn from the British Medical Association and the growing number of Royal Colleges (Saks 2003a), the allied health professions with more restricted powers also developed as the nineteenth century wore on. This is exemplified by the power gained by the GMC in 1878 to examine and register dentists, with legislation in the 1920s leading to the creation of first a Dental Board and then in the 1950s a General Dental Council, closing the profession to outsiders (Nettleton 1992). The Pharmaceutical Society of Great Britain – through Pharmacy Acts going back to the 1850s and 1860s – also won the statutory right to register pharmaceutical chemists and prevent those without qualification from dispensing medicines (Levitt et al. 1995), while the General Optical Council was established in 1958 to register ophthalmic opticians (Larkin 1983). Such allied health professions have been seen by Turner (1995) as falling into the category of 'limitation' since their operation is confined to a particular part of the body or therapeutic method. While these specific professions gained independence from direct medical supervision, they emerged as a result of medical dominance – with the sanction of the medical elite – at the cost of being enclosed within their own jurisdictions.

These occupational groups differed from the much wider cluster of allied health professions in Britain which developed in the twentieth century and are characterized by 'subordination', in which the professions in question directly took on tasks delegated by the medical profession (Turner 1995). They included nurses who are numerically the largest group in the health care division of labour. They gained professional closure through the 1919 Nursing Registration Act, which established the General Nursing Council and formalized their subordinated place under the medical umbrella (Rafferty 1996). The pre-existing medical monopoly over diagnosis and treatment also, to a considerable degree, constrained the position of the midwives who gained their professional standing through the 1902 Midwives Act (Stacey 1988). Alongside nurses and midwives – who were subsequently placed under the regulatory authority of the United Kingdom Central Council for Nursing, Midwifery and Health Visiting and then the Nursing and Midwifery Council (Davies 2002) – the professions supplementary to medicine emerged. This subordinated cluster of occupations formally effected social closure through the Council for the Professions Supplementary to Medicine in 1960 and initially consisted of boards covering chiropodists, dieticians, medical laboratory technicians, occupational therapists, remedial gymnasts, radiographers and physiotherapists (Larkin 1983). The range of such professions has now been further expanded under the less overtly subordinated badge of the Health Professions Council (Larkin 2002).

In addition to these medically dominated professions – sometimes labelled 'semi-professions' because of their more restricted remit compared to medicine – there is a wider group of health care occupations in Britain. This includes practitioners of complementary and alternative medicine (CAM) who became increasingly more marginalized with the rise of orthodox medicine from the more pluralistic system that preceded it. As such, they largely form part of the realm of 'exclusion' as opposed to 'limitation' and 'subordination' (Turner 1995). The diverse range of outlying therapies that CAM encompasses – spanning from acupuncture and aromatherapy to homoeopathy and herbalism – offered potential competition to the medical and allied health professions. Although CAM therapists were still able to practise after the mid-nineteenth century, their numbers declined steeply with the growing professional unity around the increasingly credible bio-medical paradigm in the period up to the mid-twentieth century (Saks 2005). However, spurred by the counterculture in the 1960s and 1970s, there has been a resurgence in the use of CAM practitioners by consumers. This has in part been responsible for the professionalization of osteopaths and chiropractors through the 1993 Osteopathy Act and the 1994 Chiropractic Act that established the General Osteopathic Council and the General Chiropractic Council respectively to oversee registers to oversee registers giving statutory protection of title (Saks 2006). Such practitioners, though, are currently the exceptions that prove the rule – for while groups like acupuncturists have formed voluntary registers with a view to professionalization, most still lie outside mainstream health care in the private sector (Saks 2003a).

Such non-professionalized CAM therapists in fact are a subset of the wide span of health support workers and form by far the largest element of the health care workforce in Britain (Saks 2008). Some of this workforce are becoming more professionalized, such as operating department practitioners who are now registered as a profession with the Health Professions Council (Saks and Allsop 2007b). However, it mostly incorporates wholly non-professionalized groups to whom work is sub-delegated – for instance, health care assistants, who have taken on the more menial work from nurses, and groups like foot aides and darkroom technicians, who work under the authority of chiropodists and radiographers respectively (Saks 1998). Similarly large groups of non-professionalized health support workers also exist in the United States, where the early professionalization of nursing, for example, led to registered nurses establishing a pecking order including licensed practical nurses and nurses' aides (Freidson 1970). While the existence of the latter groups highlights the extent of the subordinating influence of the health professions on both sides of the Atlantic, our focus here remains on the leadership challenges posed to the more powerful and dominant professionalized elements of the workforce in health care.

Perspectives from the United States of America

In the United States the dominance of the medical profession developed later than in Britain and was based on more fragmentary arrangements, in which there was specific legislation around the turn of the twentieth century regulating physicians in each state – thereby creating geographically distinct jurisdictions (Saks 2003a). Unlike in Britain, therefore, the closure of the American medical profession derived from a series of state licensing boards typically composed of a majority of medical society representatives. The construction of such boards was heavily driven by the American Medical Association, which was formed in the mid-nineteenth century (Starr 1982). In this system professional exclusion was based on a more formal legal basis, with competitors able to practise only if they gained separate state licences in their particular field – and even then there was no guarantee of being able to gain access to hospitals or the right to prescribe drugs, which further limited competition in the marketplace. However, among other things, the impact of the 1910 Flexner Report restricting the number and quality of medical schools meant that there were more similarities than differences in the local regulatory requirements for medicine in the United States – and by extension also between the form of exclusionary closure effected by the British and American medical profession (Berlant 1975).

Although there were threats to the autonomy of physicians in the more privatized and unco-ordinated American health care system throughout the twentieth century, there was no doubting their power and dominance – which was accentuated by the rapid growth of medical specialization on a far wider scale than in Britain, overseen by the Council on Medical Education of the American Medical Association and the related Advisory Board for Medical Specialties (Stevens 1971). Other health professions like dentists and optometrists were restricted in so far as they were simply given an exclusive licence to practise in their specific field – paralleling the sphere of 'limitation' in the British case (Freidson 1986). The power of the American medical profession, as in Britain, was especially great in relation to other allied health professions. The licensing boards were pivotal in controlling the allied professions in particular states, in association with the national Council on Medical Education responsible for accrediting non-medical university health programmes (Krause 1996). Organized medicine successfully lobbied state legislatures for the approval of licensing laws that ensured that occupations such as nursing, physical therapy and occupational therapy were also subject to 'subordination'. As such, their members could usually practise only under the supervision of a physician, a point that was typically underlined in practice contexts.

While licensed nurses in the United States managed more rapidly to develop advanced and specialized training programmes in the face of medical dominance than their counterparts in Britain (Kalisch and Kalisch 1995), midwives declined in number as they were increasingly squeezed out by obstetricians from state licensing – often becoming excluded CAM practitioners in states otherwise well served by physicians (Saks 2003a).

Although it was technically illegal to do so, a range of other CAM therapists also practised following their proliferation in the more open and aggressively democratic health care field of the nineteenth century in the United States (Porter 1992). This resulted in a greater number of CAM groups achieving exclusionary closure and at an earlier stage than in Britain. Osteopaths gained licensure in most states by the 1950s in the more liberal American political climate, albeit typically at the price of medical incorporation. In addition, the chiropractors won widespread state licensure by the 1980s, a decade before their counterparts in Britain (Wardwell 1994). While restrictions on hospital access and drug prescribing have sometimes continued to place CAM therapies at a competitive disadvantage to the medical profession, strong consumer demand has resulted in further selective state licensure of CAM groups – not least in naturopathy and acupuncture, usually on limited and/or subordinated terms (Cohen 1998).

Although the dominance of the American medical profession over other health professions has generally remained, there have been ongoing turf battles which, as in Britain, have led to encroachment on its territory. An example of this is the decline of physician representation on state licensing boards for the allied health professions, and the selective taking over of such functions as drug prescribing by nurses and pharmacists (Krause 1996). However, the greatest erosion of its power has been through the development of the role in health care of private corporations, which has long constituted a challenge to organized medicine (Saks 2003a). In the private sector physicians have been under great financial pressures to limit costs, which has impinged on their autonomy and authority. In the public sector too, significant constraints have been imposed at federal, state and local level – as illustrated by the establishment of Diagnostic Related Groups linked to Medicare (Krause 1996). This contrasts to some degree with Britain, where the medical profession has not faced a private corporate challenge on the same scale and has proved highly adept at accommodating to changes threatening its exclusionary position (Saks 2003a). Despite these variations, the medical profession has generally retained its monopolistic and pre-eminent position in the health care division of labour in both the United States and Britain.

This raises the question of how far has the leadership in medicine and the allied health professions in these countries promoted the interests of clients and the wider public in managing the issues of power and dominance in health care?

Altruism, leadership and the health care professions

Notwithstanding their differential legally defined power base, centred on social closure, most professions, from veterinary surgeons to engineers, have tended to present themselves through their codes of ethics as serving the client and/or the public interest on both sides of the Atlantic (Freidson 2001). This is certainly the position in relation to the legal profession – and has also been very apparent in the classic case of medicine and the allied health professions. The British Medical Association, for instance, has long argued that it promotes the common good and the American Medical Association equally emphasizes its commitment to service to humanity (Saks 1995). As such, they commonly draw on the altruistic aspect of the spirit of the Geneva Code of Medical Ethics, adopted by the World Medical Association (Campbell 1984), which are paralleled by the codes of ethics of nurses and other health professions that highlight their respect for human rights (see, for example, McHale and Gallagher 2003). The main differences between the codes adopted by professions in the United States and Britain, including the wider health care field, is that those in the more privatized environment of the former place greater stress on the relationship between professionals and their clients, while those in the more state-oriented milieu of the latter – particularly from the twentieth century onwards – also tend to accentuate the public responsibility of professional groups (Saks 1995).

These positive ideologies were initially accepted at face value in studies of professions in the Anglo-American context, particularly as trait and functionalist writers – who were dominant in the period up to the 1960s – tended to see professions as being based on unique bodies of specialized expertise of great importance to society (Millerson 1964). The trait approach focused on the construction of lists of the perceived distinctive attributes of professions, such as high levels of skill and altruistic service, rather than identifying such mechanisms by which to achieve exclusionary closure (see, for example, Greenwood 1957; Wilensky 1964). The more theoretically inspired functionalist perspective centred on explaining the origin of the regulatory controls giving rise to the privileges of professions in terms of the smooth functioning of social systems rather than competitive group interests. Professional groups, according to this perspective, were given their relatively high social and economic position in exchange for non-exploitative control of esoteric knowledge that is important to society (see, for instance, Goode 1960; Barber 1963).

The notion that the leadership of the health care professions has at least in part been oriented towards the service of the public is borne out by the more positive aspects of the professionalization process, such as the development of nursing as a profession in Britain. Among many other things, this paved the way for the disentanglement of nursing from the repressive hospital system that restricted the training of nurses in the late nineteenth and early twentieth centuries – as well as significantly raising the credentials of nurses in serving the wider society as the twentieth century unfolded (Witz and Annandale 2006). Writers such as Etzioni (1969) in the United

States have contentiously argued that the semi-professional standing of nursing resulted from functional processes related to the lesser need for expertise in this field as compared to that of medicine. However, the relative autonomous, if subordinated, standing that emerged through the profession-alization of nursing can be seen as a major testimony to its leadership in the politics of health care. Abel-Smith (1960) certainly sees the 1919 Nursing Registration Act as a very significant political achievement following the 'thirty years war'. In this struggle, Mrs Bedford-Fenwick set up in 1887 the British Nurses' Association, which campaigned for a state-sponsored system of registration and a Central Nursing Council responsible for the nurse training curriculum and examinations run by nurses. As part of this process, the leaders of this body skillfully used royal patronage and the regulatory precedent of midwifery to achieve their ends, while realistically ceding dominance to the predominantly male, higher status medical profession. The extent of the achievement of its leadership is underlined by the fact that nurses around the turn of the century had largely working-class origins and predominantly female gender in a patriarchal society in contrast to the generally higher status, male doctors (Witz 1992), a point noted by Bishop in her Introduction to this book.

The success of the nursing leadership in Britain was paralleled in the United States by the case of physiotherapists in the early decades of the twentieth century, whose lobby enabled the field to develop beyond the few orthopaedic surgeons in private practice who employed women with a limited amount of instruction in massage and corrective exercise, and the handful of lay assistants used by medical electro-therapeutists. In this respect, Dr Harold Corbusier astutely used his military contacts following the First World War – in which hundreds of women were trained as 'reconstruc-tion aides' on short courses – to launch the American Women's Physical Therapy Association in collaboration with Mary McMillan in 1921. This body paved the way for physiotherapy. A critical factor in its success was the acceptance of subordination to doctors (Larkin 2000). In addition to the positive impact of leadership on the successful development of professional projects, a number of other historic and contemporary examples can be given of leadership in the health care professions where such groups have used their elevated positions to the benefit of the public.

Such positive leadership includes medicine, nursing and other health professions acting as champions against potentially harmful practices in support of advances to assist patient care. In medicine, this was very apparent in the fight of the British Medical Association from the 1880s onwards against 'secret remedies', which required particularly dogged leader-ship. In its long struggle to ensure that the contents of the ever-growing numbers of patent medicines available to the public were printed on the labels of such medicines, the leaders of the British Medical Association published exposures of the composition of certain types of these remedies in the *British Medical Journal* and elsewhere – highlighting the dangers to the public of taking them (Vaughan 1992). This was exemplified by the use of everything from morphine-based soothing syrup for children teething to blue dye and caustics for the treatment of cancer, in many cases at the expense of seeking more effective medical care. Such action ultimately led to a Select Committee focused on patent medicines and foods being set up in 1912 and a welter of legislation restricting activities in this field in the first half of the twentieth century – which, among other things, limited both the advertisement and sale of remedies for such medically treatable conditions as venereal disease and the employment of substances like opium and cocaine in them (Larkin 1995).

Admittedly, this campaign could also be seen to be motivated by self-interest of groups such as doctors and pharmacists in restraining competition, especially given the scale of the multimillion pound patent medicines industry covering every kind of condition (Saks 2003a). However, the leadership offered by the British Medical Association in this field was still generally to the public good – even if it led to the enhancement of the power, status and income of the medical profession (Saks 1995). Similar claims might also be made about the struggle of the American Medical Association against 'quack' remedies in the first half of the twentieth century. The attack by the leaders of the American Medical Association on a broad range of alternative therapies via medical journals and other mechanisms was also made in the name of protecting the public. Its campaign was launched against such groups as naturopaths using toxic vitamins with negative effects and those hawking the drugless treatment of obesity through exercise and diet (Burrow 1963). However, such was the breadth of the venomous public education campaign against allegedly 'deluded' and 'deranged' charlatans – which continued in the lobby against 'cultist' and other marginalized practitioners in the second half of the twentieth century – that it is more of an open question whether the leadership offered by organized medicine was wholly in the interest of their clients or the wider public as opposed to physicians themselves (Saks 2003a).

Notwithstanding the inevitable debates about what is in the public interest in health care (Saks 1995), the case of nursing in the United States provides two good examples of where the leadership of health professional bodies can be seen to be acting for the public good in a more contemporary context. In a situation where patient care appears to have deteriorated significantly in face of corporate cost-cutting pressures in the more privatized American hospital system (Weinberg 2003), nursing associations have recently shown their leadership qualities in fighting back against such measures. At national level, the leadership of the American Nurses Association has striven to combat these trends by supporting the so-called 'Magnet hospitals', which have a good record of nurse retention, by giving them a special designation through its newly established American Nurses Credentialing Centre. At state level, nursing associations like the Massachusetts Nurses Association have taken a lead by lobbying for, among other things, legislation to ensure minimum registered nurse-to-patient ratios and to mandate more nurses for patients who need intensive nursing. Although the effects of such ratios on the flexibility to adjust the skill mix of the health care team can be debated, they at least set a tangible baseline for care (Gordon 2005).

Such campaigns also involve potential conflict with the medical profession given their impact on its interest position in the health care division of labour (Larkin 2000). This is illustrated further in Britain by the development of allied health professional groups like dentists (Thorogood 2002) and clinical psychologists (Pilgrim 2002) where boundary issues with medicine have been a focus. Stacey (1992) has nonetheless argued that – despite the imperialistic tendencies of medicine – a strong and independent contemporary medical profession has value in so far as it can speak for the health of the wider public, in acting as a buffer between the individual and the state. In her words:

> A major advantage from the public point of view of a strong and united profession is that it can oppose government proposals or actions when necessary in the interests of the health of the people ... The theory and practice of medicine has had many beneficial consequences. The power of the professions ... has, from time to time, been pitted against reactionary proposals, for example to make abortion laws more restrictive ... Scientific pronouncements of epidemiologists have drawn attention to deficiencies in the government's public health policies ... with regard to salmonella, listeriosis, nuclear power and waste.
>
> (Stacey 1992: 258)

This underlines the general benefits of strong leadership in the health professions in the broader Anglo-American context – in which professional self-interests are often subordinated to the public good. However, as Stacey herself recognized, there is a dualism to professional leadership in health care in so far as professional power can also frequently be used in a conservative and self-interested manner. In this sense, it is important from a leadership standpoint that health professions are not simply put on a pedestal and seen as altruistic groups of experts acting rationally to protect the public – as they tend to be in trait and functionalist approaches.

A more critical view of leadership in the health care professions

Since the 1970s a more critical stance has been taken towards professional groups by the social sciences, and concerns expressed about the ways that these groups have used their power more to the benefit of their own interests than those of the public. These criticisms initially took their steer from the interactionists who argued that the concept of professionalism was a socially negotiated label and the ideologies of professions – including the professional altruism ideal – could not therefore be taken at face value (Becker 1962; Hughes 1963). This was followed by broader critiques of professional bodies from a variety of perspectives. Marxist critics tended to see professions as upholding bourgeois interests in the capitalist order which prevent them from effectively serving the public, not least in the health and social welfare field (Esland 1980; Navarro 1986). Foucauldians meanwhile challenged emancipatory views about scientific progress based on the expertise of professions, highlighting the disciplinary rather than altruistic focus of their activities in such areas as psychiatry and obstetrics (Foucault 1973; Arney 1982). For our purposes though, the discussion centres on the neo-Weberian approach to professions – based on the politics of competing group interests in the marketplace – which underpins the more critical recent social scientific approach to the professions. This approach particularly underlines the leadership challenges of power and dominance in health care.

From a neo-Weberian perspective, leadership driven by self-interested groups in health care at the expense of the public may be best illustrated historically by the manner in which medicine in Britain obtained professional standing in the mid-nineteenth century before knowledge of health could substantially benefit patients – some 50 years in advance of the professionalization of the American medical profession at the turn of the century. Although functionalist writers have explained the rise of the medical profession in terms of the significance of its growing scientific knowledge base to modern society (Wallis and Morley 1976), exclusionary closure was achieved long before the pharmacological revolution and other mainstream biomedical developments in Western medicine – at a time when even aseptic techniques and anaesthesia had not been widely introduced in health care (Saks 2003a). Indeed, such closure emerged in a period when hospitals were seen as 'gateways to death' and bleeding and purging were among the mainstream treatments employed by the medical profession (Porter 2002). A far more plausible explanation of the success of the medical profession in these circumstances lies in neo-Weberian accounts based on the successful leadership of the emerging profession inspired by group self-interest.

Neo-Weberians have structurally explained the professionalization of medicine in Britain in a number of ways, including in relation to the expanding middle class that provided an increased market for medical services and helped to transcend upper-class patronage in a period of rapid industrialization (Johnson 1972). However, the quality of medical leadership was undoubtedly central in achieving this, as highlighted by the difficulties in obtaining the legislation underpinning professional closure; it took 17 bills presented to the House of Commons from 1840 onwards before the 1858 Medical Registration Act was passed (Waddington 1984). Crucial to the success of the medical profession was the work of the newly fashioned medical elite in creating a more politically powerful, solidaristic medical community and fostering greater upper-class recruitment to medicine in developing its professional standing (Johnson 1972). In this process, the leadership by key figures in bodies such as the Provincial Medical and Surgical Association, which later became the British Medical Association, in lobbying Parliament about the dangers posed by the lack of regulation was critical. So too was the astute manner in which these leaders ideologically countered liberal attacks on corporate monopolies by not formally seeking to preclude unregistered practice in health care (Saks 2003a).

Parallel comments could be made about the way in which the leaders of the American medical profession gained licensure across the range of states by the early twentieth century. Here the fragmentation of the clientele and upper-class recruitment seem to have played a similarly facilitative role in the process of professionalization (Starr 1982). It was also important for the American Medical Association through strategic leadership to gain public support for its cause, together with the sponsorship of political elites (Freidson 1970). In this respect, Berlant (1975) has emphasized that the success of organized medicine in both Britain and the United States depended on its tactics of competition as well as the socio-political conditions in which it found itself. In the United States in particular he suggests that the American Medical Association enhanced its position by exploiting the tension between national and local economic interests in face of the anti-trust movement – as it was politically vital that the monopolies encouraged through state licensure protected local economic interests against the threat of national corporations and bureaucratization. The other main difference from Britain in this context was that professionalization in the United States took place when it was easier to justify on the grounds of the development of the biomedical paradigm – even if its payoffs were still unclear in an era before drugs such as antibiotics and surgical advances had entered the picture (Saks 2003a).

Although the stage at which the professionalization of medicine occurred in the United States might be seen as less problematic from the standpoint of the public good than in Britain, it can still be viewed as being driven by self-interests in terms of the enhancement of the income, status and power of the medical profession (Starr 1982). Some of the specific tactics of its leaders in the professionalization of American medicine also seemed to be linked to group self-interest, with questionable public benefit. A good example is the way in which physicians allied with the homoeopaths in the late nineteenth century to set up state licensing boards in the United States. The collaboration was engendered by the fact that physicians seemed unable to gain licensing restrictions on their own, had linkages with the homoeopaths on the ground, and feared the effects of open warfare with such practitioners – whose relatively safe, highly diluted preparations were very popular with consumers at the time (Saks 2003a). However, once medicine had reaped the benefit of this alliance, the homoeopaths were effectively outflanked and driven virtually out of existence with the implementation of the Flexner Report in the early twentieth century. This led to the closure of almost all the homoeopathic training schools – thereby restricting the supply of physicians and eliminating a major element of market competition for the newly forged medical profession (Kaufman 1988).

Following the establishment of the medical profession in the United States and Britain, there are many critiques by neo-Weberian contributors of its leadership in the Anglo-American context for pursuing self-interest at the expense of the public interest. Thus, Johnson (1972) in Britain has argued that:

> The emergence of a succession of subordinate 'professions auxiliary to medicine' in Britain is the history of how physicians have been able to define the scope of new specialized medical roles, and cannot be regarded as ... a product of the most rational utilization of human resources.
>
> (Johnson 1972: 35–36)

To be sure, Johnson himself can be criticized for the lack of evidence adduced for this claim, which is designed to show how the leaders of professions such as medicine can impose role definitions perpetuating their own dominance at the expense of the rational application of knowledge. This view, however, deserves to be treated seriously – as it has been supported at least in part by subsequent empirical work, such as that by Larkin (1983) which considers in more detail the development of specific allied health professions like physiotherapy and radiography in the context of a dominant medical profession.

In the United States, moreover, Krause (1971) has challenged the degree to which leaders in medicine and other professional fields serve the public interest by highlighting the way in which professional power has been employed to disenfranchise the 'have-nots'. This has certainly been reflected, for instance, in the substantial differences in doctor–patient ratios between specific states in the United States. These are far greater than parallel geographical inequalities in Britain and tend to be more positively correlated with the economic and social attractiveness of these states than their incidence of ill health (Saks 2003a). This position was for long exacerbated by the resistance of the leadership of the American Medical Association to increase the number of physicians, as it was not in the financial or other interests of doctors to do so (Friedman 1962). Nonetheless, there has been a significant rise in physician numbers from the 1970s onwards as medical specialization has grown and medical schools have been substantially re-warded for increasing their throughput (Krause 1996).

Nor do such claims about the negative influence of professional self-interests on leadership in health care just relate to doctors as the dominant health care profession. They also extend to the leaders of nursing and other allied health professions. Historically, the decline of the experienced but untrained 'old wife' who attended most of the childbirths of the urban poor and lived in with their families was directly related to the legal restrictions established by the lobby for the formation of the midwifery profession in Britain in the early twentieth century (Chamberlain 1992). Beattie (1995) meanwhile has highlighted the counterproductive effects of 'tribalism' on all levels of health care leadership in contemporary Britain – which he believes has impeded inter-professional research, education and practice in the health professions. Such boundary conflict based on professional self-interests is well illustrated in the United States by the opposition of the American Nursing Association and dozens of local nursing associations in the late 1980s to the attempt by the American Medical Association to develop a new grade of registered care technologist, who would train and practise under the authority of physicians (Weiss 1997). Registered nurses themselves, more-over, have had their own boundary disputes with unlicensed nurses in the United States, precipitated by the managerial pressures for cost containment (Brannon 1996).

Whatever the potential longer-term gains from such turf battles, they have negative implications for relationships in health care. The negative effects of health leadership – or rather the comparative lack of it – are no better highlighted than in relation to recent public concerns about the regulation of health care professions in Britain. While there has been reform of all the major health care professions in the UK since 1997 to ensure greater lay engagement and accountability, there are still major concerns about the limited protection offered to the public – especially from incompetent doctors by the self-regulating medical profession through the GMC (Allsop and Saks 2002). This was underlined by the case of Dr Harold Shipman, the general practitioner who went undetected for many years despite killing at least 250 of his patients, and a number of other recent medical scandals – such as the unacceptably high rates of child heart surgery at Bristol Royal Infirmary and the removal of organs from deceased children without consent at Alder Hey Hospital in Liverpool (Allsop 2002). These events prompted the recent reviews by Donaldson (Department of Health 2006a) and Foster (Department of Health 2006b) covering medicine and the wider spectrum of health professions, including health support workers (Saks and Allsop 2007b). The result of these reviews has been a government White Paper enhancing professional regulatory practices, including continuous fitness to practise procedures (Department of Health 2007). This underlines how positive leadership outside the health professions can be just as important as that from within in terms of public protection – even in relation to the most powerful and dominant of such professions.

Health care leadership for the public good

This latter point is crucial as it demonstrates that leadership in driving health policy can be as significant as that in the health professions themselves in facilitating the public good – especially when the self-interests of dominant professions prevail over the public interest, notwithstanding their altruistic ideologies in the Anglo-American context. This can be exemplified further by the range of policies promoted over recent years aimed at making a positive difference to health care. These span from the establishment of the Office of Minority Health in the 1980s by the United States Department of Health and Human Services, which sought to reduce disparities in black health (Rice and Winn 1991), to the introduction by the British government of the Patient's Charter in the early 1990s, which explicitly set out the rights of patients and the standard of service to be expected from health professionals (Alaszewski 1995). Although there may be debate about their ultimate effectiveness, these health care reforms depended on proactive leadership to drive them forward – sometimes despite professional resistance. This is an issue that is highlighted in the final chapter of this book when considering how to develop leadership in the health care professions.

However, in dealing with leadership challenges in health care, it may be easier to implement change through the empowerment of the health professional groups involved rather than seeking to impose solutions from above. This is particularly the case where powerful health professional elites are involved, such as those in medicine, with self-interests in perpetuating the status quo (Huczynski and Buchanan 2007). Having said this, in some situations the interests of such groups may lie in change, with resistance to preserving existing positions – as, for example, when there are opportunities to enhance the form of professional closure to their strategic advantage. Whatever the specific position, though, effective empowering leadership may be the key to advancement where professional self-interests pull in different directions from that of the public good. Otherwise there is a real danger that professions will simply adapt in counterproductive ways to neutralize externally imposed policies. For instance, in response to the introduction of general managers in the National Health Service in Britain to effect greater control over the health professions with the Griffiths reforms of the 1980s (DHSS 1983), many doctors simply moved into these roles – thus minimizing any abrogation of their authority (Strong and Robinson 1990).

In handling the leadership challenge posed by professional power and dominance in health care, it is also important that the health professions including doctors, nurses and other allied health professional groups are constructively directed towards the public good – if necessary through suitable incentivization in relation to their interests. Here leverage may be exerted by radical subcultures within professions and consumer groups with different interest identities (Saks 2000). In this regard, developments in accord with professional interests have been conceptualized in this chapter as leading to the objective enhancement of power, status and/or income (Saks 1995). In dealing with the dynamics of self-interests and providing suitable incentives for positive action, it should be noted that such interests may not always be subjectively perceived or indeed followed by the professional groups concerned. An example of this is illustrated by the introduction of the Medicare health insurance programme for elderly people in the United States in the mid-1960s. Although this was manifestly in the interests of doctors as it increased the pool of medical fees and gave them greater freedom to increase their income through prescription and treatment, there was initially strong opposition to Medicare from many parts of the American medical profession (Moran and Wood 1993). In terms of orchestrating a positive future, therefore, the interplay of leadership, professional self-interests and the public good is a complex equation.

This complexity is made all the greater as the notion of the public good is itself an extremely slippery concept, which is often left totally undefined in political usage or simply employed by social scientists as an ideology for analysis. There are indeed many disparate definitions of this term, which take on distinctive shades in the hands of particular disciplines and writers (Saks 1995). However, it is very important that the notion of the public good is operationally defined if clear objectives and visions of the future are to provide positive direction for professional leadership (Brooks 2006). At a micro level, this concept has been taken in this chapter to relate to the individual interests of clients in enhancing their well-being – recognizing that there are some circumstances where these may conflict with collective interests, as with the need for quarantine for contagious diseases (Campbell 1984). At a macro level, the concept of the public interest has been pragmatically viewed in terms of the overarching values of the country in which it is being judged – in this case the specific framework of liberal-democratic values in Britain and the United States, based on the particular balance struck between freedom, justice and the advancement of the overall welfare in each of these societies (Saks 1995).

This analysis of leadership for the public good in relation to power and dominance in the health professions has been undertaken primarily at the macro level. However, as is acknowledged in the previous chapters, it should be remembered that leadership takes place at many levels in health care, including at a micro level – from local workplaces such as hospitals and clinics to the one-to-one interactions of health professionals with clients. At all levels there are many ways in which leadership skills related to the web of professional self-interests and the public good can be developed in the health care professions – such as through leadership programmes as described by Antrobus and her colleagues in Chapter 5, action learning sets and coaching and mentorship – including provision specifically tailored to doctors, nurses and allied health professions (see, for instance, Edmonstone 2005). In such settings particular theories of leadership can be discussed, applied and evaluated. These span from the different bases of power that can be used to influence the behaviour of key players – including the power to reward and coerce, as well as act from a basis of legitimacy and expert knowledge – to the effect that specific styles of leadership, such as the charismatic and the informal, can have on others (Huczynski and Buchanan 2007).

Conclusion

More research clearly needs to be undertaken into the leadership challenges posed by power and dominance in the health care professions and the ways in which they can be resolved using a range of research methods (Saks and Allsop 2007a). However, this chapter at least provides some insights into the dynamics of this field and how such challenges can best be managed for the public good either by or outwith the health care professions. In the particular case of nurses and the allied health professions, it provides a pointer as to how the leadership of such groups can be further empowered when the odds may be stacked against them in the power relations inherent in the longstanding, but shifting, health professional pecking order. For all health professional groups including the still dominant medical profession, the leadership challenges in health care centrally include how their members can be persuaded to consistently serve the public good in practice where this may involve them putting the public interest before their own professional self-interests.

Key points

- Health care professions in Britain and the United States, on which the chapter is focused, have a legally defined power base – with the dominant medical profession at the top of the pecking order in the wider health division of labour.
- Medicine, nursing and the allied health professions present themselves through their altruistic codes of ethics as promoting the interests of clients and/or the wider public.

- There are many cases where the leadership of the health care professions translate these ideologies into practice and serve the public, sometimes in spite of their own self-interests.
- However, in recent decades an increasing number of cases have come to light where the leaders of such professions have put professional self-interests before the public good.
- This highlights the importance of engendering positive leadership in health care to promote the interests of the public – which can be best achieved by empowering the leaders of the health professions themselves.
- There are various means through which the interests of the leaders of medicine, nursing and the allied health professions can be harnessed to the benefit of the public in meeting the challenge of professional power and dominance.

Reflective exercises

1 Consider actions in health care that can be seen to advance the public good – in individualistic and collective terms. Outline instances in particular where doctors, nurses and the allied health professions have promoted the interests of clients and/or the wider public.

2 Provide examples of occasions in which the self-interests of professional groups in health care have prevented the public good from being realized. Explore the particular challenges that power and dominance in the health care professions pose to leadership in this light.

3 Drawing upon the literature, examine the role of leadership in ensuring that situations in health care where there is a clash between professional interests and the public interest can be positively resolved.

4 Using your own experience as appropriate, reflect on the relevance of the analysis to your present or likely future position in the health workforce. How might this impact on your leadership strategy?

References

Abel-Smith, B. (1960) *A History of the Nursing Profession*. London: Heinemann.

Alaszewski, A. (1995) Restructuring health and welfare professions in the United Kingdom: the impact of internal markets on the medical, nursing and social work professions. In T. Johnson, G. Larkin and M. Saks (eds) *Health Professions and the State in Europe*. London: Routledge.

Allsop, J. (2002) Regulation and the medical profession, In J. Allsop and M. Saks (eds) *Regulating the Health Professions*. London: Sage.

Allsop, J. and Saks, M. (2002) Introduction: the regulation of health professions, In J. Allsop and M. Saks (eds) *Regulating the Health Professions*. London: Sage.

Arney, W. (1982) *Power and the Profession of Obstetrics*. London: University of Chicago Press.

Barber, B. (1963) Some problems in the sociology of professions. *Daedalus* 92: 669–688.

Beattie, A. (1995) War and peace among the health tribes. In K. Soothill, L. Mackay and C. Webb (eds) *Interprofessional Relations in Health Care*. London: Edward Arnold.

Becker, H. (1962) The nature of a profession. In National Society for the Study of Education (ed.) *Education for the Professions*. Chicago, IL: University of Chicago Press.

Berlant, J.L. (1975) *Profession and Monopoly: A Study of Medicine in the United States and Great Britain*. Berkeley, CA: University of California Press.

Brannon, R.L. (1996) Restructuring hospital nursing: reversing the trend toward a professional work force. *International Journal of Health Services* 26: 643–654.

Bratton, J., Callinan, M., Forshaw, C. and Sawchuk, P. (2007) *Work and Organizational Behaviour*. Basingstoke: Palgrave Macmillan.

Brooks, I. (2006) *Organisational Behaviour: Individuals, Groups and Organisation*, 3rd edn. Harlow: Pearson Education.

Burrow, J.G. (1963) *AMA: Voice of American Medicine*. Baltimore, MD: Johns Hopkins University Press.

Campbell, A.V. (1984) *Moral Dilemmas in Medicine: A Coursebook in Ethics for Doctors and Nurses*. 3rd edn. Edinburgh: Churchill Livingstone.

Chamberlain, M. (1992) The old wife, pregnancy and birth control. In M. Saks (ed.) *Alternative Medicine in Britain*. Oxford: Clarendon Press.

Cohen, M. (1998) *Complementary and Alternative Medicine: Legal Boundaries and Regulatory Perspectives*. Baltimore, MD: Johns Hopkins University Press.

Davies, C. (2002) Registering a difference: changes in the regulation of nursing. In J. Allsop and M. Saks (eds.) *Regulating the Health Professions*. London: Sage.

Department of Heath (2006a) *Good Doctors, Safer Patients. Proposals to Strengthen the System to Assure and Improve the Performance of Doctors and to Protect the Safety of Patients: A Report by the Chief Medical Officer* (Donaldson Report). London: Stationery Office.

Department of Health (2006b) *The Regulation of the Non-medical Healthcare Professions: A Review by the Department of Health* (Foster Report). London: Stationery Office.

Department of Health (2007) *Trust, Assurance and Safety: The Regulation of Health Professionals in the 21st Century*. London: Stationery Office.

Department of Health and Social Security (DHSS) (1983) *NHS Management Enquiry* (Griffiths Report). London: DHSS.

Edmonstone, J. (ed.) (2005) *Clinical Leadership Development*. Chichester: Kingsham.

Esland, G. (1980) Diagnosis and therapy. In G. Esland and G. Salaman (eds) *The Politics of Work and Occupations*. Milton Keynes: Open University Press.

Etzioni, A. (ed.) (1969) *The Semi-Professions and their Organization*. New York: Free Press.

Foucault, M. (1973) *Madness and Civilization*. London: Tavistock.

Freidson, E. (1970) *Profession of Medicine*. New York: Dodd, Mead.

Freidson, E. (1986) *Professional Powers: A Study of the Institutionalization of Formal Knowledge*. Chicago, IL: University of Chicago Press.

Freidson, E. (2001) *Professionalism: The Third Logic*. Cambridge: Polity.

Friedman, M. (1962) *Capitalism and Freedom*. Chicago, IL: University of Chicago Press.

Goode, W. (1960) Encroachment, charlatanism and the emerging profession. *American Sociological Review* 25: 902–914.

Gordon, S. (2005) *Nursing Against the Odds*. New York: Cornell University Press.

Greenwood, E. (1957) Attributes of a profession. *Social Work* 2: 45–55.

Huczynski, A.A. and Buchanan, D.A. (2007) *Organizational Behaviour*, 6th edn. Harlow: Pearson Education.

Hughes, E. (1963) Professions. *Daedalus* 92: 655–668.

Jewson, N. (1976) The disappearance of the sick-man from medical cosmology 1770–1870. *Sociology* 10: 225–244.

Johnson, T. (1972) *Professions and Power*. London: Macmillan.

Kalisch, P.A. and Kalisch, B.J. (1995) *The Advance of American Nursing*, 3rd edn. Philadelphia, PA: Lippincott.

Kaufman, M. (1988) Homeopathy in America: the rise and fall and persistence of a medical heresy. In N. Gevitz (ed.) *Other Healers: Unorthodox Medicine in America*. Baltimore, MD: Johns Hopkins University Press.

Krause, E. (1971) *The Sociology of Occupations*. Boston, MA: Little, Brown.

Krause, E. (1996) *Death of the Guilds: Professions, States, and the Advance of Capitalism, 1930 to the Present*. New Haven, CT: Yale University Press.

Larkin, G. (1983) *Occupational Monopoly and Modern Medicine*. London: Tavistock.

Larkin, G. (1995) State control and the health professions in the United Kingdom. In T. Johnson, G. Larkin and M. Saks (eds) *Health Professions and the State in Europe*. London: Routledge.

Larkin, G. (2000) Health workers. In R. Cooter and J. Pickstone (eds) *Medicine in the Twentieth Century*. Amsterdam: Harwood Academic.

Larkin, G. (2002) The regulation of the professions allied to medicine. In J. Allsop and M. Saks (eds) *Regulating the Health Professions*, London: Sage.

Levitt, R., Wall, A. and Appleby, J. (1995) *The Reorganized National Health Service*, 5th edn. London: Chapman and Hall.

Macdonald, K. (1995) *The Sociology of the Professions*. London: Sage.

McHale, J. and Gallagher, A. (2003) *Nursing and Human Rights*. Oxford: Butterworth Heinemann.

Millerson, G. (1964) *The Qualifying Associations*. London: Routledge and Kegan Paul.

Moran, M. and Wood, B. (1993) *States, Regulation and the Medical Profession*. Buckingham: Open University Press.

Navarro, V. (1986) *Crisis, Health and Medicine: A Social Critique*. London: Tavistock.

Nettleton, S. (1992) *Power, Pain and Dentistry*. Buckingham: Open University Press.

Parry, J. and Parry, N. (1976) *The Rise of the Medical Profession*. London: Croom Helm.

Pilgrim, D. (2002) The emergence of clinical psychology as a profession. In J. Allsop and M. Saks (eds) *Regulating the Health Professions*. London: Sage.

Porter, R. (1992) Introduction. In R. Porter (ed.) *The Popularization of Medicine 1650–1850*. London: Routledge.

Porter, R. (2002) *Blood and Guts: A Short History of Medicine*. London: Allen Lane.

Rafferty, A.M. (1996) *The Politics of Nursing Knowledge*. London: Routledge.

Rice, M.F. and Winn, M. (1991) Black health care and the American health system: a political perspective. In T. Litman and L. Robins (eds) *Health Politics and Policy*, 2nd edn. New York: Delmar.

Saks, M. (1995) *Professions and the Public Interest: Medical Power, Altruism and Alternative Medicine*. London: Routledge.

Saks, M. (1998) Professionalism and health care. In D. Field and S. Taylor (eds) *Sociological Perspectives on Health, Illness and Health Care*. Oxford: Blackwell Science.

Saks, M. (2000) Medicine and the counter culture. In R. Cooter and J. Pickstone (eds) *Medicine in the Twentieth Century*. Amsterdam: Harwood Academic Publishers.

Saks, M. (2003a) *Orthodox and Alternative Medicine: Politics, Professionalization and Health Care*. London: Sage.

Saks, M. (2003b) The limitations of the Anglo-American sociology of the professions: a critique of the current neo-Weberian orthodoxy. *Knowledge, Work and Society* 1: 11–31.

Saks, M. (2005) Political and historical perspectives. In T. Heller, G. Lee-Treweek, J. Katz, J. Stone and S. Spurr. (eds) *Perspectives on Complementary and Alternative Medicine*. Abingdon: Routledge and the Open University.

Saks, M. (2006) The alternatives to medicine. In J. Gabe, D. Kelleher and G. Williams (eds) *Challenging Medicine*, 2nd edn. Abingdon: Routledge.

Saks, M. (2008) Policy dynamics: marginal groups in the health care division of labour in the United Kingdom. In E. Kuhlmann and M. Saks (eds) *Rethinking Professional Governance: International Directions in Healthcare*. Bristol: Policy Press.

Saks, M. and Allsop, J. (eds) (2007a) *Researching Health: Qualitative, Quantitative and Mixed Methods*. London: Sage.

Saks, M. and Allsop, J. (2007b) Social policy, professional regulation and health support work in the United Kingdom. *Social Policy and Society* 6: 165–177.

Stacey, M. (1988) *The Sociology of Health and Healing*. London: Unwin Hyman.

Stacey, M. (1992) *Regulating British Medicine: The General Medical Council*. Chichester: Wiley.

Starr, P. (1982) *The Social Transformation of American Medicine*. New York: Basic Books.

Stevens, R. (1971) *American Medicine and the Public Interest*. New Haven, CT: Yale University Press.

Strong, P. and Robinson, J. (1990) *The NHS: Under New Management*. Milton Keynes: Open University Press.

Thorogood, N. (2002) Regulating dentistry. In J. Allsop and M. Saks (eds) *Regulating the Health Professions*. London: Sage.

Turner, B. (1995) *Medical Power and Social Knowledge*, 2nd edn. London: Sage.

Vaughan, P. (1992) 'Secret remedies' in the late nineteenth and early twentieth centuries. In M. Saks (ed.) *Alternative Medicine in Britain*. Oxford: Clarendon Press.

Waddington, I. (1984) *The Medical Profession in the Industrial Revolution*. London: Gill and Macmillan.

Wallis, R. and Morley, P. (1976) Introduction. In R. Wallis and P. Morley (eds) *Marginal Medicine*. London: Peter Owen.

Wardwell, W. (1994) Differential evolution of the osteopathic and chiropractic professions in the United States. *Perspectives in Biology and Medicine* 37: 595–607.

Weinberg, D.B. (2003) *Code Green: Money-driven Hospitals and the Dismantling of Nursing*. New York: Cornell University Press.

Weiss, L.D. (1997) *Private Medicine and Public Health: Profit, Politics and Prejudice in the American Health Care Enterprise*. Boulder, CO: Westview Press.

Wilensky, H. (1964) The professionalization of everyone? *American Journal of Sociology* 70: 137–158.

Witz, A. (1992) *Professions and Patriarchy*. London: Routledge.

Witz, A. and Annandale, E. (2006) The challenge of nursing. In J. Gabe, D. Kelleher and G. Williams (eds) *Challenging Medicine*. London: Routledge.

4 Leadership for the allied health professions

Mary Lovegrove and Tyrone Goh

Overview

There is more recognition across the world now than at any time in the past of the capacity of the allied health professions (AHPs) to make a real difference to the lives of patients and to develop new ways of working. Changing demands in health services aligned with fundamental changes in the organization of care delivery in the UK have conspired to highlight the broad range of AHPs' expertise and skills that previously have been somewhat hidden. However, the extent to which this workforce can significantly improve patient care is still not well understood in many parts of the world. In this chapter we highlight some of the major developments in Australia, Singapore and the UK where the AHP workforce has been empowered to provide evidence of their effectiviness in the health care team. Strategic leaders of the AHP workforce have networked within a country and between countries to share experiences and to agree collective approaches to developing and nurturing their practitioners.

Here we explore the concept of effective leadership for this diverse group of professionals; the challenge for leaders, and the significant positive impact on patient care that comes from visionary clinical practitioner and academic leaders.

Introduction

Allied health professionals (AHPs) work at different levels for different employers. These professionals work in different settings, and across many sectors, including health, education, social services, primary care, independent sector and the third sector. Many of these professionals are not employed in the mainstream health sector but are employed either by Social Services or by the Voluntary Sector. This diverse employment opportunity facilitates formal and informal networking between practitioners and departments within local authorities and other services. This ensures that the clinical protocols and care pathways for service delivery across organizational boundaries are robust.

Allied health professionals are normally graduates who are educated and trained inter-professionally with other AHP groups, and occasionally with medical students, student nurses and student midwives. The majority of AHPs are autonomous practitioners and as such are skilled as 'first contact' for the patient or client. They are used to working with complex pathways and interface with other agencies, and are familiar with positive risk taking. They are also used to helping patients and service users to take risks appropriately, in order to maximize independence, including self-care and self-management. In addition AHPs are enablers for service users, preventing inappropriate admissions, reducing length of stay in hospital and reducing delayed transfers of care. Increasingly the significant contribution this group makes to service delivery and health and social care is being recognized across the world. Services must respond to the changing health needs of the population and individual communities. Patterns of ill health have altered since the mid-twentieth century, with the trend moving towards higher incidence of stress-related and lifestyle-influenced conditions and increasing numbers of people living with long-term illness (Scottish Executive 2005a).

The concept of allied health professions: some global perspectives

The concept of allied health professions is well established and relatively well understood in some countries and less well in others. Australia has led on the development of a recognized identity for allied health groups, and in the late 1980s championed the emergence of the 'allied health' workforce and the importance of strategic leadership for this group. Historically, allied health in Australia has been viewed – as in most Western countries – as allied to medicine. However, more recently it is considered in a collaborative context, leading to the need to clarify the issue of how most effectively the allied health workforce can deliver the service (Boyce 2006). The Allied Health Professions Australia (AHPA) is the national lead body for key health professions and their representative bodies, and significantly, does not include representatives of medical practitioners, nurses or health care unions. Recognized by the Australian government at federal and national level, the

AHPA is the voice of the allied health professions sector on all political and strategic issues. Uniquely, the allied health sector in Australia has an additional network for those working in rural and remote locations, with membership of the rural and remote committee including those covered by the Australian allied health workforce and representatives from social work and pharmacy.

Following the political stance of their Australian colleagues, the Canadian Health Professionals Secretariat (CHPS, which represents 60,000 allied health professionals across Canada) drew to the attention of the newly formed Health Council of Canada a report which set out the progress on health care renewal and the health status of Canadians. The Council in turn published a report in 2004 highlighting the integral role that allied health professionals play in health care delivery, and outlined the problems created by staff shortages (Canadian Intergovernmental Conference Secretariat 2004). The report supported the voice of the CHPS in acknowledging that the human resources crisis and its impact on patient care extends well beyond doctors and nurses.

Similar difficulties in the provision of quality health care, in particular the input of AHPs in their contribution to care, have arisen in the United States, where the impact of health care reforms has resulted in dramatic changes in the manner by which health services are delivered. Organizational, legal and financial structures have been transformed in much of the US health care services into systems of integrated care that combine primary, specialty and hospital services. The goal of these new systems was to reduce costs, to improve health care outcomes, and to enhance consumer satisfaction. It was projected that the concomitant loss of many hospital beds, and the expansion of primary care into ambulatory and community settings would require the re-engineering of the careers of many of the allied health professionals. Across the Atlantic these changes are echoing in the UK, where since the mid 1980s, each of the four countries, England, Northern Ireland, Scotland and Wales, have been seeking solutions to demographic and economic dynamics. Each of the four countries has a named Health Professions Officer, who, as the senior government adviser on allied health professions issues provides a leadership focus, albeit a government-led one – as is the case in nursing.

The NHS Scotland in particular has championed the development of the allied health workforce. Clinical leadership has been identified by the Scottish Executive as crucial to supporting the change process and is reflected in the NHS Scotland Leadership Development Framework (Scottish Executive 2005b). AHPs are encouraged to capitalize on available opportunities that inter-professional and inter-agency working provide so that they build their leadership capacity and foster clinical leadership skills at all levels. Involvement in, and leading, health improvement initiatives and developing new and extended roles in the management of long-term illness, are areas where

AHP leadership skills seem certain to bring significant benefits in the coming months and years. The Scottish Executive has also highlighted the importance of succession planning and sustainability of new roles in the AHP-led modernized service.

The NHS in England is divided into 10 strategic health authorities (SHAs) which are responsible for managing the local NHS. According to the SHA Allied Health Professions Leads for England, the term allied health professional relates to arts therapies (art, music, drama and play), chiropody and podiatry, dietetics, occupational therapy, orthoptics, paramedics, physiotherapy, prosthetics and orthotics, radiography (diagnostic and therapeutic), speech and language therapy. This workforce is over 130,000 strong with the majority of its members regulated by the Health Professions Council in the UK. Many also elect to become members of their uni-professional bodies, for example the Society of Radiographers, the College of Occupational Therapists. Some of these professional bodies have, in turn, linked with similar professional bodies in other countries to form international societies, such as the World Federation of Occupational Therapy, The International Society of Radiographers and Radiological Technologists. These international bodies are formally recognized by the World Health Organization and by the European Union. The chief executives of the UK professional bodies have joined together as a co-operative to form an influential body called the Allied Health Professions Federation (AHPF). The role of the AHPF is to provide leadership to member professional bodies and to influence government policy, and is singularly placed to make sure that health, social care and education decision makers understand the unique contribution of the allied health professions.

The professional developments in nursing in Hong Kong described in Chapter 1 have paved the way for further development in the allied health professionals' education. In 2007 the Hong Kong Hospital Authority launched its Institute of Advanced Allied Health Studies. This is an all-inclusive organization which supports the development of the qualified practitioner across the allied health workforce and other related professional groups. The Hospital Authority in Hong Kong refers to an extended allied health family which includes all the professions identified in the English Strategic Health Authority AHP leads list (as mentioned above) and in addition it includes audiology, clinical psychology, medical physics, medical laboratory technology, medical social work, optometry and pharmacy.

Similarly, in Singapore, the Ministry of Health has placed a focus on allied health professionals be they therapists, podiatrists, radiographers or radiation therapists. They have realized that there is a personnel shortfall of these professionals and have taken steps to increase the graduates from the local polytechnic for physiotherapists, occupational therapists, radiographers and radiation therapists. For the other AHPs, where training is not available in the local institutions of higher learning, they have increased the number of scholarships for pre-qualifying degrees to study speech therapy, psychology, podiatry for example in established universities in the United Kingdom, Canada, the USA and Australia. The Ministry of Health also increased funding to support public hospitals to pay for additional staff, which in turn will enable senior allied health professionals to focus on upgrading and training their junior staff. Protected time is also given to those who are interested in teaching and research, and scholarships are awarded to them to pursue their Master's degrees and doctorates. A further initiative by the Ministry of Health in Singapore to boost staffing levels has been the establishment of an accreditation committee to review overseas qualifications, so that those who qualify will not face delays from the immigration and personnel ministries.

The reasons for the acute shortage of allied health staff in Singapore are the rapid expansion of health care facilities in Singapore, and the government's anticipation of the increase in the numbers of elderly patients between 2008 and 2020 (Ministry of Health 2008). With this in mind the Ministry has also commissioned a publicity company to create new and interesting information via the media on the roles of the allied professionals, to encourage more potential students to these professions. The local television station has even directed a television series depicting them in the hospital setting. The Ministry of Health, in collaboration with the public health care groups, have completed a salary benchmarking exercise and has reviewed and revised the salaries of AHPs in 2007 and 2008 to ensure that the public sector salaries of AHPs are as competitive as those in the private sector. With the advances in medicine, and in keeping with the United Kingdom and Australia, the Singapore government has realized that a diploma as an entry qualification to the allied health profession is not sufficient and they are, at the time of writing, exploring the idea of a university course for the professions. Of the graduating cohort who hold a diploma, 95 per cent have pursued further study to upgrade their qualifications to a degree by studying degree conversion programmes offered by universities in the United Kingdom and Australia.

Supporting the need for leaders within the AHPs, the Ministry of Health in Singapore invites some of their members to join many decision making committees pertaining to their professions, services and career pathways, positions previously taken by either senior doctors or administrators on behalf of the AHPs. Experts in various AHPs are also members of committees involved in providing services for the ageing population, those with chronic diseases and those delivering primary health care. To show support to the AHPs, ministers and senior politicians are gracing events organized by the professional societies. With the advent of role expansion, the government has called on AHPs to evaluate and redefine whether their role is current with those of developed countries. As with nursing, many AHPs have risen to the challenge and are in dialogue with the Ministry on expanded roles, for example, radiographers have been encouraged to explore their role in reporting of plain X-ray examinations and certain radiological procedures. To ensure that members of the public are protected, the Ministry will also be initiating the state registration of AHPs, similar to that of doctors, nurses and pharmacists. In terms of career advancement, AHPs in Singapore are doing relatively well as many have been placed in senior management positions, some holding senior posts in hospitals and institutions such as chief executive officers and executive directors or general managers. Therapists are also employed as Directors of Operations or Head of Allied Health, indicating that the health care institutions are recognizing the capabilities of these professionals in management and leadership roles. *This development, which should be transferable across countries, can be sustained only if the leadership potential for the united AHP workforce is released.* Historically AHP services have been organized and led by uni-professional managers with little transdisciplinary activity. This situation is beginning to change with the gained wisdom and insight into the potential for a multidisciplinary approach.

The collective AHP approach

Dr Rosalie Boyce, an advocate for the collective AHP voice, argues that contextually organizational models are central to the success of the impact of the AHP strategy and decision making process (Boyce 2006). Significant influence of AHPs can happen only if the historical position of tribalism is rejected and the professionals readily accept the stronger collectivist model of the Allied Health Professionals. Beabout et al. (2001) argue that collectivism is the theory and practice that makes the group the fundamental unit. They further postulate that views of the groups are more important than those of the individual members.

There is extensive debate about AHPs. Are they a group of separate individual professions (a federation), or do they have a professional identity distinct from other similar groups such as doctors and nurses? AHP leaders across the world have to come to an agreement about this position and to decide whether they represent a newly identified collective profession or a collection of disparate groups. The current debate is polarized as to whether the patient's view of the AHPs is leading the argument or the position taken by the professional discipline. If the leaders of AHPs operate from a position of collaborative care for a greater number of patients, rather than from a position of an individual profession, they then have a right to view collectivism as the ideological path. However, there is a real risk if the rights of individual professions supersede those of collective groups if the larger individual professions believe that they have a greater right of say. The argument that 'we have the largest membership and as such we are the highest priority' can be damaging to a collectivist philosophy, which in essence means equal rights for all groups irrespective of size. Such debates link well with the work of Saks in Chapter 3, where professional protectionism is highlighted. Some philosophers argue that forests do not exist but only trees. Clearly forests do exist and the impact of a large forest such as a rain forest is well known. The leaders of allied health professions must see the workforce as a forest rather than a group of separate trees. Once this consensus is reached we will be able to optimize the collective impact of the AHPs. What remains to be identified is the group identity and the collective rights of that group. A consequence of this approach is the perceived risk to the individual profession and the perceived immoral under-valuing of the smaller groups. However, the counterargument is the empowering of the minority groups through the combined strength of the collective.

Today there is more recognition than at any time in the past of the capacity and capability of the AHPs to make a real difference to the lives of patients and to develop new ways of working (Department of Health 2008). Allied health professionals perform essential diagnostic and therapeutic roles within health and social care. They perform the functions of assessment, diagnosis and treatment throughout the care pathway from primary prevention through to specialist disease management and rehabilitation using applied science. Working with individuals from all age groups and within all clinical specialties, their particular skills and expertise can be the most significant factor in helping people to develop and maintain their independence through both physical and mental rehabilitation. A unique contribution of AHPs is their ability to meet the combined mental and physical health needs of service users. It is also recognized that AHPs will have a major contribution to make to the newly emerging care pathways such as stroke care, cardiac care and end of life care and models of care delivery such as polyclinics and local hospitals. AHPs can play a key role in providing the full spectrum of care for patients and carers from primary prevention through to specialist disease management and palliative care. It is increasingly recognized that AHPs are in an excellent position to challenge the existing organizational structure and influence any change that is required to improve the patient experience. However, to maximize this AHPs must demonstrate their cost-effective contribution that their specialist skills can make to improve the health and well-being of service users and their carers. This is an opportunity for AHPs to take advantage of their transferable skills in order to lead service change. They should make explicit the contribution they can make to improve a person's quality of life through reducing their reliance on services and by promoting health and well-being.

Frameworks for change

In 2002 the Department of Health in England launched the 10 key roles for AHPs. They continue to be the reference point for the leaders of these practitioners. Set out in Table 4.1 are the agreed statements relating to each of the 10 key roles (Department of Health 2002a).

Table 4.1   Allied health professionals' 10 key roles

1	To develop extended clinical and practitioner roles which cross professional and organizational boundaries.
2	To be a first point of contact for patient care, including single assessment.
3	To diagnose, request and assess diagnostic tests, and prescribe, working with protocols where appropriate.
4	To provide consultancy support to others promoting the AHP contribution to patient independence and functioning, training, developing, mentoring, teaching, informing and educating health care professionals, students, patients and carers.
5	To develop extended clinical and practitioner roles which cross professional and organizational boundaries.
6	To manage and lead teams, projects, services and case loads, providing clinical leadership.
7	To develop and apply the best available research evidence and evaluative thinking in all areas of practice.
8	To play a central role in the promotion of health and well-being.
9	To take an active role in strategic planning and policy development for local organizations and services.
10	To extend and improve collaboration with other professions and services, including shared working practices and tools.

AHP career pathways

The AHP career pathways are numerous, flexible and diverse. The key leadership pathways are clinical leadership, strategic leadership and academic leadership. The clinical leadership career pathway is the most complex with graduate clinicians becoming specialists, specialist generalist and/or extending their scope of practice. The consultant allied health professional is the highest grade with responsibility for a clinical caseload, education and research leadership.

AHPs populate all levels of the strategic leadership pathway, from therapy managers to chief executives of health care organizations, however, the number of AHPs holding these very senior posts is still relatively small, but increasing. Similarly in education, leadership AHPs are heads of academic departments, dean posts through to vice chancellors. Academic leaders benefit enormously from engaging and guiding the education and training of this wide and diverse professional group. They are enabled to increase their knowledge, skills and competencies and assume greater responsibility for working with clinical AHP leads to develop innovative responsive clinical services and the education and training to support the new developments. In the UK the modernization and redesign of clinical and education services enables AHP careerists to pursue an expanded career pathway, with increased job options and potential for increased job satisfaction. An example of such an opportunity will be the AHP clinical academic posts. Here they will become actively involved in multidisciplinary research and the identification of outcomes which will be integrated into the future planning and provision of clinical services and skills audit, ensuring that learning from research and audit is implemented into care pathway development initiatives.

The AHP leader and developing AHP leadership

Leadership for Allied Health is more than 'managing' the service (see Chapter 2), more than being a 'therapy lead' – it is about leading the staff and subsequently the service to a new position. This requires an in-depth understanding of all the constituent parts, all the traditions and cultures that accompany the existing professional structures and professional values. It requires strength of character and determination to follow a realistic long-term vision and to expect and anticipate that along the journey there may be extensive opposition, challenges and barriers to achieving the goal to enhance patient care. To be a leader in one of the disciplines requires courage and tenacity as well as the ability to communicate the vision effectively (Paterson 2008). To be an effective leader for allied health, the individual needs all the leadership skills expected of any professional leader and also the exceptional skills of considered negotiation and articulated respect for the knowledge and skills of the mix of disciplines they lead.

So often critics query how somebody from a different discipline could lead them or even understand the service that they deliver, or their professional needs. Inspirational allied health leaders will succeed through evidence of sustained achievement, and will themselves take on a new generic allied health identity. Over time they will adapt to embrace the skills and values of the wider AHP community that they lead, as distinct from adhering to uni-professional behaviour. They will continue to challenge the status quo and to lead and further develop the service for the benefit of the service user (patient and/or student). Nonetheless, it is essential that true AHP leaders should aspire to maintain their original clinical identity, not only to support and enhance the opportunities for the professional discipline, but also to support individuals through senior professional networks. Other professionals such as nurses, who have chosen to relinquish their original professional status, have lost peer respect and are criticized for leaving behind the core values and clinical expertise of their profession (see Chapter 7).

Effective leadership is central to the success of providing a modern and responsive service (Institute for Innovation and Improvement 2006). This is particularly important for AHPs given their range and diversity. Successful leadership requires a focus on developing and maintaining effective relationships at all levels within the organization and with other relevant external partners. It is about empowerment and setting oneself and one's services up to succeed. Managers may or may not have good leadership skills to be an effective leader. This point is discussed in detail in Chapter 7, where Stanley identifies the tensions between management and clinical leadership. He makes the point that clinical leadership comes from hands-on care, from maintaining clinical expertise and may, at times, be somewhat divorced from management. In our view effective leadership is less about pushing the way forward but more about pulling the clinical team behind you when you have a clear vision; it is about leading people through transformational change to develop better services for the local community. There are significant opportunities for AHPs to be more involved in strategic decision making within the local health economy, nationally and internationally; and to translate strategy into operational delivery; to lead on significant pieces of work, such as long-term care; and to promote the development of integrated teams. AHP leaders should exist at all levels and across all sectors, and should be recognized and identified as key players. They should capitalize on available opportunities that inter-professional and inter-agency working provides so that they build their leadership capacity. AHP clinical leadership skills at all levels is crucial to support any change process. Integrated AHP leadership capacity at board level has already demonstrated the effectiveness of integrated working across the professions in supporting organizational priorities (Department of Health 2000).

To be an effective AHP team leader it is essential that the individual understands that being an AHP team leader is often broader than simply being responsible for one organization or team and that no team can stand alone. As mentioned earlier, many of the staff they lead may express concern that the leader could not possibly understand their discipline specific needs and peers may see them as representing only the discipline that they trained in; it is the AHP leader's responsibility to demonstrate a non-partisan approach to their work, and this can be achieved only through a clear understanding and acceptance of the unique position of the lead allied health professional as distinct from the uni-professional leader. There is a widely held view that supports findings of the US National Commission on Allied Health, which identified inflexible curricula and disciplinary boundaries as the principal barriers to change in professional education (Leja and Wardley 2002). The Commission recommended that higher educational institutions should reduce compartmentalization of health professions, and introduce interdisciplinary training, and enhance collaboration between programmes. The positives of inter-professional learning are perhaps overridden by the breadth of knowledge required by all health care workers, and the need for each discipline to develop its own research – based expertise. This issue is discussed more fully later.

The quality of AHP leadership is not consistent – but then neither is it in other disciplines. There are some exceptional individuals at the top but they are too few. Successful AHP leaders have a vision for their organization which transcends short-term issues and targets. They are passionate about high performance and high quality in their organizations, and they are also authentic and good at communicating to staff and those around them. They understand the climate and culture in their own organization and in the wider health and social care environment. Many of the AHP professional bodies issue guidelines for professional clinical leaders (College of Radiographers 2005) and actively encourage the development of advanced and consultant practitioners, advocating that advanced practitioners should act as an expert resource and should provide effective leadership for an area or section of the service taking account of the relevant legal, ethical and professional frameworks. The professional bodies also expect the consultants to promote and contribute to development of effective integrated care teams and provide professional leadership. These posts normally carry an education and research role as well as the responsibility for advancing the clinical service for the benefits of the patients.

An example of a very successful innovation is that provided by a consultant musculoskeletal physiotherapist. The reason that the innovation described in Case study 4.1 has been so successful is not only because it has been shown to be an excellent response to service need, but also because it was led by a highly motivated and committed expert practitioner. The practitioner concerned has a high degree of personal professional clinical autonomy and is well regarded by medical and non-medical colleagues as an evidence-based leader in this field.

Case study 4.1 Clinical leadership by a consultant musculoskeletal physiotherapist

Musculoskeletal triage for physiotherapists was developed in response to a redesign in service provision at a University NHS Trust in England. In 2006 there were a thousand patients on the waiting list for musculoskeletal outpatients' physiotherapy. The longest wait had risen to 42 weeks and the physiotherapists were normally assessing the patients, for 40 minutes before beginning a course of treatment.

The consultant musculoskeletal physiotherapist, who is jointly employed by the Trust and University, redesigned the services so that the most experienced clinicians could triage all new patients in 20 minutes before deciding on the most appropriate form of physiotherapy intervention.

The consultant physiotherapist then developed an education and training programme and taught the experienced clinicians the skill of adapting the 40 minute assessment to a 20 minute triage appointment. Just one year after starting this new service, the patient waiting time for musculoskeletal triage had been reduced to four weeks.

To change the service in this way the consultant physiotherapist demonstrated all the traits and competencies needed to be a leader: an effective leader and communicator who motivates and inspires others to deliver optimum quality of care within the specialist field and beyond. The practitioner is an acknowledged resource of expertise and was able to challenge current structures and identify organizational and professional barriers which limit/inhibit services and provide solutions to overcome them.

Previously in order to progress their careers, frontline allied health professionals such as this consultant physiotherapist would have had no choice but to dispense with the clinical side of their work and take on a more managerial role. *It is essential that those working closest to patients make significant improvements to patient's care, eradicate outdated practices and overcome institutional barriers.*

Therapists in all specialists are now taking direct referrals from general practitioners (GPs), running clinics and fast-tracking patients. For example consultant podiatrists have surgical podiatry skills and are able to treat patients with orthopaedically compromised feet as well as having extensive knowledge of high-risk foot conditions. These skills enable the establishment of services to treat patients with high-risk problems as a result of diabetes, vascular insufficiency or rheumatological problems as well as requesting imaging procedures.

Increasingly senior clinical allied health professional practitioners are running the services that have previously been led by medical practitioners. This further strengthens the partnership between the expert practitioner and the patient. An example of such a development is the consultant therapeutic radiographer who runs the gynaecological oncology service (see Case study 4.2). This development has received national (UK) recognition. The post-holder is convinced that the success of this development is based on effective leadership through the identification of a need for change and commitment to introduce new ideas in an 'environment of resistance'. The post-holder advises that an emphatic approach to managing change and enhancing the ideas of team ensures better outcomes for the patient, and acknowledges that communication at all levels and valuing all members of the team can enhance the working relationships and encourage individual development and contribution to better health care service.

Case study 4.2 Role of consultant radiographer in gynaecological oncology

The position of consultant radiographer in gynaecological oncology was established in March 2005. Prior to this development the post-holder had been employed as an advanced practitioner in therapeutic radiography. Initially the role was established with the expressed aim of improving the service to women undergoing brachytherapy treatment for gynaecological tumours. The specific remit was to review and audit the current practice, to review the information available to the patients and to evaluate their support post-treatment. As the role evolved it became evident that there was an opportunity to identify areas of change that could positively impact on the cancer patients' journey and overall patient outcomes.

Following bespoke training, development of competency packages and Trust agreed protocols the vaginal vault brachytherapy service was transferred from a medical-led service to a service led and run by a radiographer. This resulted in patients being able to undergo the procedure as a day case admission rather than an overnight stay. The outcome was improved patient satisfaction, reduced inpatient costs and greater service efficiency.

This development resulted in considerable interest by the Macmillan Cancer Support Charity. They agreed to fund this consultant practitioner post subject to the development of a comprehensive psychosexual support package for the patients. The research to inform this publication has commenced. Phase one will evaluate the patient compliance with the dilator used for treatment compared to the national standard. Phase two will involve in-depth interviews with women who have undergone pelvic radiotherapy. The aim is to understand how we can better deliver information on the use of vaginal dilators and sexual health. The output will be a comprehensive education tool designed and influenced by women which will then inform national practice hopefully leading to better patient compliance.

Challenges for AHP leaders

It is recognized that all leaders face challenges on a daily basis (NHS Confederation 2007), however, the AHP leader has some very specific challenges. Normally the individual has experience of leading a uni-professional team but little or no experience of leading a diverse multiprofessional team with a range of service deliverables. Often the constituent groups operate from a different philosophical paradigm and have very different value sets. The membership of the collective group will determine the leader's response to managing the wider team. Organizations should strategically release the leadership potential in their staff and support AHPs to add value through working in effective clinical teams. This could be achieved by creating new Head of Allied Health posts with the stated responsibility to lead – as well as manage – a collective allied health workforce. To attract and retain inspirational leaders to these posts the organizations will need to consider line management of these individuals to empower them to influence and steer the clinical teams to deliver an enhanced patient service.

Many of these groups will deliver their services on a traditional historical model and a key challenge for the AHP leader is to understand the service boundaries to enable any service redesign based around patient experiences. For inter-professional engagement the leader must be understanding and sensitive to diverse viewpoints and they must be able and prepared to lead staff to the position where commitment and loyalty is to the delivery of the patient-led service, rather than to a particular team or organization. Sometimes there is dissonance between the needs of patients, clients and service users and the delivery of the effective service based on organizational convenience. It is the responsibility of the AHP leader to be tenacious and challenge this position to model an agreed acceptable way forward. For an effective merger of traditional services there is the risk of resistance, cultural clash, with the inevitable reliance on organizational structure. The challenge for the leader is to develop a coherent culture and a united approach to working practices.

There is evidence (Hughes 2007) that strong leaders and champions are needed for change, particularly in inter-professional teams. The concept of an AHP workforce is truly inter-professional and without that understanding

AHP leaders will not succeed. For effective AHP leadership the leaders must have shared inter-professional values and clarity of direction. The shared values are ones that all colleagues irrespective of professional discipline can share and should be developed during the initial education and training period. Chapter 6 in this book deals comprehensively with future education requirements for health leaders of the future, and the authors underline that the clarity of direction will be influenced by political drivers. However, these can only be fully understood when there is an agreed collaborative culture to enable true inter-professional working to take place. AHPs have a long record of working in multidisciplinary teams, working across organizational boundaries and providing shared services, and are well placed to be regarded as a key resource for inter-professional learning, involving users and carers in service design and development and in creating effective multiprofessional partnerships.

The numbers of experienced AHP leaders internationally are relatively few as yet, and there is no recognized international network to support this increasingly important group. There are a number of local and national networks emerging, their structures often reflecting the way that AHP services are managed. Currently there are too few clinical AHP leads and identifying role models is a recognized challenge. Often the post-holder is identified by their professional discipline rather than as a key leader across the AHP spectrum. Finding capacity to clinically lead a new multi-professional team is a significant problem for many AHP leaders as the organizational structures may not have adjusted sufficiently to enable a carefully planned development programme to be followed.

Modern health care systems require leaders to undertake significant transformational change rather than just incremental changes to achieve the desired results. An example in England is the shift of focus of service delivery from the traditional acute model to patient-led community-based services. The government recognizes that AHP leaders are central to successful realignment of services across the eight key areas of care (Department of Health 2007). These are:

- Maternity and newborn care
- Children's health
- Planned care
- Mental health
- Staying healthy
- Long-term conditions
- Acute care
- End-of-life care.

This review of the NHS requires all AHPs to review their working practices. Historically many therapists have worked a standard week and the therapy care has been left to the staff remaining in the hospital or there has been in gap in the service. Clinicians have suggested that sustained AHP care and patient support throughout the week results in improved patient outcomes for those with long-term rehabilitation needs. AHP leaders should support management in building flexibility within existing working patterns and budgets by adopting a range of strategies to minimize gaps in service and ensure continuity by implementing proactive approaches to recruitment, planned leave and staff turnover. AHP leaders should aim to incorporate elements of capacity planning to reflect organizational priorities. For example many patients with long-term conditions have an improved quality of life when they have access to rehabilitation therapy outside of the traditional working week. This requires developing a new rehabilitation therapy workforce possibly at assistant or associate practitioner level able to work in a rehabilitation department or on a stroke or long-term conditions ward. This workforce has a range of skills enabling them to take actions to provide a seamless service to patients with proximal supervision from a registered AHP practitioner or rehabilitation nurse. They undertake a range of delegated tasks and delegated authority and report to a registered practitioner. These rehabilitation therapy assistant or associate practitioner roles are successful where an infrastructure of support is present and the function, competencies and accountability of the roles have been clearly thought through and discussed. It is essential that the role redesign is seen as an integral part of the service redesign. For effective implementation, there must be support from the allied health leader, role identification in the strategic plan and clear unambiguous role specification to ensure effective teamworking (Lovegrove and Pratt 2009). Without these features in place the leader will have difficulty managing the expectations of new staff and existing staff.

AHPs can develop their leadership potential, develop and extend the existing AHP roles, and also create new roles to deliver a new service. To enable this to happen AHPs must be prepared to be proactive, be prepared to change and not to be precious about their personal professional discipline. They are often accused of complaining about their situation, they comment that organizations are not inclusive and do not recognize their transferable skills. AHP leaders must be more overt in demonstrating their extensive skill base as other professional groups are very willing to take on the responsibility for representing AHP views, and leading the AHP services. Other professionals' willingness to take on the role of AHP services leader does not mean that they understand the cultural environment in which AHPs work and the breadth of expertise that they can offer.

Robust AHP networks can empower the AHP leaders to work together effectively, share best practice and provide a very supportive environment. An example of a recent AHP network development is the London AHP leaders' network (see Figure 4.1). Until April 2007, the NHS structure for

London consisted of five independent strategic health authorities, the largest of which was the North East London. In 2003 the Chief Executive Officer of the North East London Strategic Health Authority was persuaded by two AHP leads, one the clinical AHP lead, for a mental health trust and an occupational therapist by profession and the other an AHP academic lead and a radiographer by profession, to review the organization operational structure. Their aim was to ensure direct allied health professions input to the strategy and operation of the North East London Strategic Health Authority sector. The outcome of these discussions was the establishment of an identified lead AHP post for that strategic health authority. The newly appointed postholder set up an AHP leads network, including a monthly AHP leads forum, for North East London Strategic Health Authority (NELSHA).

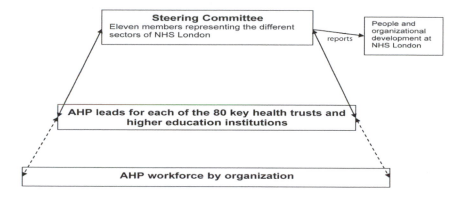

Figure 4.1   suggested London AHP Lead communication structure

In 2006 it was announced that the NHS London would be reviewed and that as of April 2007 there would be one Strategic Health Authority for London (NHSL). The AHP lead for NELSHA called an informal meeting of the local SHA AHP leads and invited other key AHP leads from the other four sectors. The group shared their concern about the need for a clear pan-London communication strategy for AHPs, and agreed to informally establish a lead AHP group for London. Since then there have been a number of workshop events for the lead AHPs for London, and a London focused agenda. The NHS London in turn has formally recognized that the AHPs should be recognized as a group in their own right and has agreed to administrative support for the AHP leads steering committee. The AHP leads for London are active in all aspects of the NHS London reforms. They have direct AHP representation on all key committees. The AHP workforce for London is some 17,000 strong with 80 key Allied Health Professional leads across the province. The communication network between the NHS London and AHP workforce is facilitated and supported by a pyramidal shaped communication model. One of the members of the steering committee of the lead AHPs for London is London's representative on the Health Professions Officers' advisory forum. This is a model that would transpose across regions, offering support and opportunities for would-be leaders to connect with each other and to share the wider agenda.

Allied health professionals as leaders of the clinical service

Fundamental to the delivery of the health service is careful attention to AHP workforce capacity and capability. A key objective to supporting the delivery of health and social care priorities is to ensure that there are sufficient numbers of trained, motivated AHPs working in the right locations (Scottish Executive 2006). There are also challenges and opportunities in terms of changing working practices and liberating the talents and skills of the AHP workforce so that every patient gets the right care in the right place at the right time (Department of Health 2005). As with all health care professionals AHPs have a responsibility for ensuring that they provide evidence-based clinical services, and that these services have clear professional and managerial accountability structures. In order to exercise their responsibilities, it is vital that AHPs are integral to the communication networks, and have equitable access to information systems, clinical supervision and continuing professional development. Evidence exists that AHP leaders demonstrate a commitment to the development of evidence-based clinical services and a commitment to management decisions (Department of Health 2002b). It is important for organizations responsible for health services such as primary care trusts (PCTs) to appreciate and to harness the contribution that AHPs can make to achieve the local and national performance targets. Furthermore, it is vital that AHPs understand what performance targets *they* are being measured against and are able to influence these targets to ensure they are outcome-based and meet agreed standards. AHP leaders can work together to address lengthy waits for patients and service users across priority care groups, in particular children's and diagnostic services in line with current and future targets. Skilled clinical leadership skills bring significant benefits to the health improvement initiatives particularly in developing new and extended roles in the management of long-term illness. Ideally a whole systems approach to care pathways should be used to support the development of specialist and consultant AHP roles within the clinical team and a process should be in place for evaluating the contribution of these roles. For example the PCTs should ensure the development of skills for all AHPs, including negotiating and influencing skills and business planning and service development skills, so that the engagement of all internal and external stakeholders is maximized. Additional challenges are posed for the PCTs as the AHP services are delivered through a shared service, cross-agency and independent contractor arrangements. Because of this cross-agency working AHPs are well-placed to highlight and to lead the modernization of some of the hidden blockages in the system, such as waits for community-based equipment which can compromise the service as a whole and the client has a less than optimum overall experience.

This is an exciting time for AHP leaders, with huge opportunities to inform the planning of services that are designed to tackle health inequalities and social exclusion, and promote health improvement. They already work in and across integrated health and social care teams for both primary and secondary services. They are the obvious leaders for designing and supporting patient care pathways and for improving access through flexible delivery with a plurality of providers. AHPs need to use their expertise to influence and shape the future health service. There is evidence that AHP-led service redesign initiatives have reduced waiting times and improved access across the United Kingdom (Department of Health 2008). AHPs already know and value the benefits of working in partnership with patients, carers, other professions and care agencies and have expertise in a range of assessment, diagnosis, treatment and rehabilitation interventions that can be more fully exploited in health terms.

Leadership in allied health through education

Traditionally health professional programmes of education in the UK were run from uni-professional schools such as schools of physiotherapy or schools of speech and language therapy. With the transfer of these schools into higher education there have been opportunities to explore ways in which the pre-registration allied health education and training can be coalesced to facilitate greater understanding of each other's roles, and where there is potential for duplication. Inter-professional learning for health is strongly advocated as it is believed that it will encourage better teamworking in practice. It is clear from the reports from the Bristol Inquiry (Kennedy 2001), the Victoria Climbié Inquiry (Laming 2003) and the Shipman Inquiry (Smith 2003) that the lack of inter-professional working and communication was fundamental to the tragic outcomes. It has been suggested by many health professionals and educators that introducing students to inter-professional learning at an early stage may be an effective way of avoiding problems in practice (Health Education Academy 2005; Kerrell et al. 2008). Clinicians report that students educated alongside students from other professional disciplines demonstrate good teamworking abilities as qualified practitioners and can work well in multidisciplinary teams within the clinical environment.

On this evidence many allied health uni-professional departments have merged into larger academic departments of allied health sciences. At the core of the modern pre-registration allied health programmes is the inter-professional learning. Academic leaders for allied health know that for effective inter-professional learning the academic staff have to share the vision and understanding of the value of this approach to learning, and ensure that inter-professional learning for allied health is not seen as merely replicating multiprofessional teams that might exist in practice. It is important to capitalizing on the academic setting to provide a forum for critical debate, discussion and learning about how allied health staff can work together and learn together with respect and understanding of differences. AHP academic leaders know the value of bringing the staff of the academic disciplines together and of fostering an academic environment of trust and enquiry so that narrow perspectives and professional academic tribalism is actively discouraged. This can best be achieved through a multiprofessional working environment in the higher education institution. Students educated and trained in this environment have a greater understanding of the perceptions and stereotyping that impedes inter-professional work. There is no guarantee that academics working in a truly inter-professional setting will be advocates for inter-professional learning. This presents the allied health academic leader with additional challenges in aiming to strategically guide the students learning experience towards that of a multidisciplinary allied health team player with a unique specialist set of clinical competencies as determined by the service and the areas of care.

Clinical allied health leaders of the future will benefit enormously from the inter-professional education leadership for allied health that has developed since 2000, when the higher education institutions were challenged to design inter-professional pre-qualifying programmes of study; however, the students are faced with understanding the mixed messages they receive from the allied health practitioners. Many practitioners will argue that the only learning that matters is the clinical expertise to deliver the patient care from the discipline specific perspectives, others will encourage the inter-professional learning, recognizing its potential to improve patient care and reduce the risk of repetition for the patient.

Conclusion

The idea of an allied health professional workforce is increasingly becoming accepted as a particular collective with a shared organizational structure and shared values and goals. However, there is still considerable debate about the focus of this workforce and there is more work to be done to reach a global consensus.

AHPs work across many sectors including health, education, social services, primary care, independent and voluntary sectors. To be an effective AHP team leader it is essential that the individual understands that being an AHP team leader is often broader than simply being responsible for one organization or team and that no team can stand alone. In order to achieve this there is a pressing need to release the leadership potential of the AHPs in a measured and informed way, through careful planning and development of the AHP workforce.

All health professional leaders need to look beyond traditional methods of providing services and engage in service redesign and role development. This will enable them to develop existing patterns of working and create new models of service that reach across historical professional and service boundaries for the benefit of the patient/client/service user. Much of the criticism of the AHP workforce has suggested that it is lacking in the confidence and support to influence real improvements in patient care within their wider health economics. The case study offered from Singapore provides an excellent example of how AHP leadership could integrate more with policymakers. The suggestion that AHPs (and other professionals), need to maintain a narrow discipline identity has led to silo working in some areas, with many AHPs identifying more with their profession than their organization, or the wider health care community. While each professional should be very aware of their discipline's contribution to health care, the need to influence care within a collaborative concept is vital if the maximum potential of care is to be realized.

Key points

- Leadership in the allied health professions is key to maximizing the potential of AHPs in health care services.
- AHPs must make and take opportunities to influence policy at all levels.
- Leadership is not a uni-disciplinary responsibility.
- AHPs are, by the nature of their work in cross-professional working, versatile, with the capability to adapt and respond to changing demands.
- Leadership in allied health can be nurtured through inter-professional education and training.

Reflective exercises

1   Using your own experience and drawing on the literature, reflect on the advantages and disadvantages of multidisciplinary working for effective leadership for allied health professionals.

2   Spend some time reflecting on the various leadership skills employed by the allied health professions. Reflect on your preferred leadership style for effective leadership of a multidisciplinary team.
3   Reflect on how strategic leadership for the allied health professions workforce is provided in your country. Compare your own experience with that of similar practitioners in another part of the world and identify what changes you would make to improve effective strategic leadership for this workforce.

References
Beabout, G.R., Swan, K., Paffenroth, K., Crespo, R.K., Grabill, S.J. and Gronbacher, G. (2001) *Beyond Self-Interest*. Lanham, MD: Lexington Books.

Boyce, R. (2006) Using organisation as a strategic resource to build identity and influence. In R. Jones and F. Jenkins (eds) *Managing and Leading in the Allied Health Professions*. Oxford: Radcliffe.

Canadian Intergovernmental Conference Secretariat (2004) *First Minister's Meeting on the Future of Health Care*: www.hc-sc.gc.ca.

College of Radiographers (2005) *A Framework for Professional Leadership in Clinical Imaging and Radiotherapy and Oncology Services*. London: College of Radiographers.

Department of Health (DoH) (2000) *Meeting the Challenge: A Strategy for the Allied Health Professions*. London: DoH.

Department of Health (2002a) *Bulletin for Allied Health Professionals – November, England*. London: DoH.

Department of Health (2002b) *Managing for Excellence in the NHS*. London: DoH.

Department of Health (2005) *Liberating the Talents: A Strategic Framework for Allied Health Professionals and Nurses*. London: DoH.

Department of Health (2007) *Our NHS, Our Future: Interim Report, England* (Darzi Report). London: DoH.

Department of Health (2008) *High Quality Care for All: The Next Stage Review, Final Report, England* (Darzi Report). London: DoH.

Health Education Academy (2005) *The Theory–Practice Relationship in Interprofessional Education*, Occasional paper no. 7. London: Higher Education Academy Health Sciences and Practice.

Hughes, L. (2007) *Creating an Interprofessional Workforce Programme: An Education and Training Framework for Health and Social Care in England*. NHS South West: www.institute.nhs.uk/
index.php?option=com_mtree&task=viewlink&linkid=3088&Itemid=165.

Institute for Innovation and Improvement (2006) *NHS Leadership Qualities Framework*. London: NHS Institute for Innovation and Improvement.

Kennedy, I. (2001) *Learning from Bristol: The Report of the Public Inquiry into Children's Heart Surgery at the Bristol Royal Infirmary 1984–1995*. London: Stationary Office.

Kerrell, R., Kitchen, S., Lovegrove, M., Sidhu, S. and Holder-Powell, H. (2008) *New Models for Learning for Allied Health Professionals: An Evaluation of the Expectations and Experiences of Clinicians, Students and Academic Staff. End of Study Report*. London: King's College London and South Bank University.

Laming, W. (2003) *The Victoria Climbié Inquiry*. London: HMSO.

Leja, J.A. and Wardley, C.S. (2002) Future trends in health care doctoral education. *Journal of Allied Health* 31(4): 227–231.

Lovegrove, M. and Pratt, G. (2009) *The Good Practice Guide: Negotiated Curriculum Design and Co-delivery National Vocational Qualifications and Foundation Degrees.* London: NHS Widening Participation in Learning Unit.

Ministry of Health (2008) *Broadening, Deepening and Transforming Health Care,* Publication 114:09/28–5 Singapore: www.moh.gov.sg/mohcorp/speeches.aspx?id=19780.

NHS Confederation (2007) *The Challenges of Leadership in the NHS.* London: NHS Confederation: http//networks.csip.org.uk/_library/

Paterson, A. (2008) Aiming high. *Synergy News.*

Scottish Executive (2005a) *Building a Health Service Fit for the Future – National Framework for Service Change in the NHS in Scotland.* Edinburgh: Scottish Executive.

Scottish Executive (2005b) *Delivery through Leadership: NHS Scotland Leadership Development Framework.* Edinburgh: Scottish Executive.

Scottish Executive (2006) *Allied Health Professions Workload and Management.* Edinburgh: Scottish Executive.

Smith, J. (2003) *The Shipman Enquiry:* www.The-Shipman-Inquiry.org.uk.

5 Developing political leaders in nursing

Sue Antrobus, Annie Macleod and Abigail Masterson

Overview

Despite international commitment to improving their political expertise (ICN 2002), nurses in all countries of the world continue to experience difficulties accessing and influencing local, national and international political agendas. Why is this? If nurses are to influence emerging health systems they must be equipped with the right skills and knowledge that will enable them to act decisively and successfully within the realms of policy and politics. In this chapter we describe the results of an independent evaluation of a programme devised to develop political leadership ability. The findings demonstrate the impact of the programme; participants gain confidence in their ability to engage with, lobby and influence politicians and policymakers and develop a more sophisticated understanding of how policy is influenced and how political institutions work.

Introduction

The literature suggests that nurses and nursing could, and should, be more engaged in shaping policy to improve health, but little has been written about how to prepare nurses to influence policy effectively, or the knowledge and skills required for effective political leadership. Here we will explore how one national nursing association (NNA) is developing political leadership capacity in its members through enabling them to lobby on key policy priorities.

Shaping patient-centred health policies that are clinically relevant, and that aim to improve public health, is an essential component of nursing leadership, yet internationally nurses face challenges accessing the political arena and contributing successfully to policymaking processes. The International Council of Nurses believes that NNAs have a responsibility to influence health policy. One of the ways in which the political profile of NNAs can be raised is through improving their members' political expertise.

This chapter derives from the findings of five annual independent evaluations of a programme devised and run by the Royal College of Nursing (RCN) in the United Kingdom. The Political Leadership Programme aims to develop the political leadership capability of its members around national lobbying priorities that have been identified by the RCN. The evaluation sought to explore participants' experiences and stakeholders' perceptions of the programme, in addition to the impact of the lobbying activity undertaken by the participants. The results of these collective evaluations, while exploratory in nature, offer a valuable insight into the development of political leaders in nursing and how a political leadership programme can increase nurses' engagement with policymakers and politicians. They suggest that NNAs should invest in political leadership programmes to encourage the development of nursing as an effective lobbying force.

Background

Nurses in all countries of the world continue to experience difficulties accessing and influencing local, national and international political agendas (Hennessy 2000; West and Scott 2000; Maslin-Prothero and Masterson 2002; Antrobus 2003).

The reasons for this are multiple and complex. Although nurses have a wealth of expertise and experience to offer to the policymaking process, this expertise is frequently overlooked by policymakers who often view clinical staff as limited in their knowledge of the broader issues that impact upon population health and service delivery. Nurses, in turn, tend to view policymakers as divorced from clinical and practical reality. Influencing policymakers and politicians requires a language that spans both practice and policy and demonstrates the impact that policy decisions will have on both populations and individual patients.

Nurses mostly deal with individual patients and use language associated with patient needs. Yet, to be effective in policy circles, nurses need to be able to construct strong arguments that relate both the patients' perspective, and clinical realities, to political debates. Nurses have minimal exposure to the study of health policy during their pre-registration programmes and do not, in the main, invest in their own development as political leaders once qualified. If nurses are to influence health policy and systems they must be equipped with the right skills and knowledge that will enable them to act decisively, and successfully, within the realms of policy and politics.

This chapter opens by offering a brief review of the literature on political leadership and political leadership programmes. The background to the establishment of the RCN Political Leadership Programme is discussed, and its aims, content, format and structure are outlined. The methods used to evaluate this programme are described and a summary of the findings presented. Finally, the implications for nurses and NNAs internationally are examined.

Political leadership: insights from the literature

The term political leadership is most commonly associated with local government and elected officials, only latterly has the term been used by professional groups operating within the public sector to describe the shaping and influencing of policy (Rafferty 1995; Antrobus 2003).

Kotter and Lawrence (1974) studied elected mayors in the US and identified three facets of political leadership: the setting of policy, its execution, and organization and service management. Game (1979) examined political leadership in UK local government and highlighted three areas as being important: agenda setting, task accomplishment, and network building and maintenance. More recently, Leach and Wilson (2002) developed the following framework to describe how political leaders work: maintaining cohesiveness; developing strategic direction (internal); representing the authority in the outside world (external); and ensuring programme implementation. There are no such descriptions of the processes and outcomes of political leadership in nursing.

The nursing literature in the UK, with a few exceptions, namely Taylor (1995), Antrobus and Kitson (1999) and Antrobus (2003, 2004) tends to consist of rallying calls for nurses to get involved in policymaking (Masterson and Maslin-Prothero 1999), but offers little in the way of practical examples about how nurses might achieve this, or the leadership skills that are needed to do so. Antrobus (2003) suggests that nurses, as political leaders, can deliver improved health outcomes for patients and communities by creating and influencing policies in ways that take into account their experience of caring for patients, the research evidence and the perspectives of those that use the service.

Although all nursing roles have a political dimension and all nurses need to be politically aware, not every nurse aspires to political leadership. The difference lies in the level at which nurses are choosing to work. Just as all nurses need to be research aware, not every nurse aspires to be a researcher.

Leadership takes place within three overlapping domains, and these are explored in further detail in Chapters 2 and 7:

- Clinical leadership
- Strategic/executive leadership
- Political leadership.

For the purposes of this chapter we are focusing on the political domain. Being politically aware, for clinical leaders, involves sophisticated political skills to implement policy, influence strategically inside their organization, and translate evidence into improvements in practice. Political leadership involves translating the evidence and experience of caring for patients into solutions that are primarily concerned with improving public health in its widest context.

Although not everyone aspires to become a political leader in nursing, the skills of political leadership are arguably becoming increasingly important for nurses at the clinical level who are expected to be involved in multi-agency and inter-professional work and in strategic work to implement national and regional policy (see Box 5.1).

Box 5.1 Political leadership: a framework of skills and knowledge

- Identifying the right issue for policy change – *whole systems thinker*.
- Mapping a constituency and developing a collective voice – *facilitator and enabler*.
- Moving the issue from the tactical to the strategic and developing strategic objectives – *strategic thinker*.
- Identifying stakeholders and mapping their positions in relation to your issue – *political operator*.
- Constructing different messages for different stakeholders using evidence and experience – *articulate speaker*.
- Building and using networks for influence – *influential operator*.
- Negotiating coalitions and aligning common goals – *collaborative worker*.
- Reviewing learning and evaluating strategic objectives – *reflective thinker*.

The skills of politics are learned – but nurses have a head start if they can start to apply their nursing skills and knowledge in new ways.

Another way of looking at the different locations of political activity is Mason *et al.*'s (2002) four spheres. They describe the four spheres of the workplace, government, professional organizations, and the community. This is arguably more useful to nurses who want to become politically aware, because it opens up alternative ways in which nurses may have a voice, which is not limited to professional channels. The four spheres emphasize the interdependence of the different arenas; they open up opportunities for all nurses, even those who may feel they have limited scope for influence in their workplace, and still have an important and influential role to play in other spheres, such as the community.

In the UK, health service delivery is inescapably political as each successive government has sought to pursue different political agendas through the National Health Service, with profound impacts on nurses and nursing, as has been noted in Chapter 1. An analysis of the political impact of nursing as a collective body has been conducted in the United States. Cohen et al. (1996) identified four stages in the development of political leadership in nursing:

- *Stage 1*: 'buy in' is where the profession recognizes the importance of political activism.
- *Stage 2*: 'self-interest' is where nursing develops and uses its political expertise as it relates to the profession's self-interests.
- *Stage 3*: 'political sophistication' is where the profession goes beyond self-interest and recognizes the importance of activism on behalf of the public.
- *Stage 4*: 'leading the way' is where the profession provides what they term as true political leadership on broader health care issues in the public interest.

We would propose a fifth stage, **global leadership**, where nurses assume an international political leadership role enabling coalitions to form that bring about action on issues of health, social and humanitarian concern to countries and communities. Internationally, interest in political leadership in nursing is growing. In the United States there are courses (see, for example, Buerhaus 1992), internships and fellowships in policy and politics that can be accessed by nurses. The American Nurses Association runs workshops to develop the political leadership skills of nurses. The Canadian Nurses Association (CNA 2000) has described how nurses can prepare for political action. Ehlers (2000) stresses the importance of united political action for nurses in South Africa to ensure nursing stays relevant to the political realities of the country and its people. The International Council of Nurses (ICN) has a Leadership for Change Programme which, although not specifically focused upon political leadership, does include health planning and policy development (ICN 2002). In addition, nursing journals regularly publish interviews with nurses working in government bodies and high profile figures in NNAs.

A search of the Athens, British Nursing Index, CINAHL, ASSIA, JSTOR and SOSIG databases, using 'politics', 'policy' and 'leadership', revealed little literature on the impact of political leadership programmes. In social science the literature focuses on 'real' political leaders and their impact, for example Presidents, Members of Parliament and local councillors (see for example Hambleton 1998; Bell et al. 1999; Siegel 2001; Leach and Wilson 2002). In nursing the literature tends to be restricted to evaluations of the components of pre-registration curricula designed to raise students' political awareness (Taylor 1995) and post-registration clinical leadership initiatives which contain elements of political awareness (Cunningham and Kitson 2000; Woolnough and Faugier 2002). An evaluation of the ICN's Leadership for Change Programme indicates that its impact at regional and national policymaking levels was variable (ICN 2002).

The RCN Political Leadership Programme (PLP)

The Royal College of Nursing Political Leadership Programme (RCN PLP) aims to prepare nurses to work effectively at a policy level. Focused on influencing government policy the PLP teaches nurses *how* to exert policy influence through taking forward a 'live' issue in a way that has direct impact on politicians and policymakers. The 'live' issue will already have strategic relevance for the RCN and its specialist groups, including a constituency of support among the membership and may already have been debated at RCN Congress.

Delivered annually, as part of the service the RCN offers to members, the programme enables a cohort of up to 24 active members to learn how they can work at a national policy level to influence and achieve policy change. A number of key interventions are used, which combine structured input and specially designed tools, with experiential learning approaches grounded in the participants' activity with the RCN.

Delivered over 12 months, with 6 days' attendance, the PLP supports nurses, through political mentoring, and coaching in political processes. Master classes include sessions on the nature of political leadership and policymaking with access to a range of international expertise including politicians, political leaders, policy and media commentators and lobbyists. Workshop activity then focuses on identifying and analysing stakeholders, constructing influencing strategies, building effective coalitions, communicating messages with vision and impact and experiencing government.

The programme supports nurses, through political mentoring, and coaching in political processes, to identify and then put into action a political issue that is 'live' for the RCN and its membership. The RCN's political networks are capitalized upon to enable participants to access the policymaking arena. The aims and outcomes of the programme are outlined in Box 5.2 below.

Box 5.2 Overall aims and learning outcomes of the UK Political Leadership Programme

Primarily focused on influencing health and social policy this action-orientated programme uses a range of innovative learning techniques and draws upon well-established political networks to enable health care practitioners to

- Influence the policy agenda to secure intended outcomes
- Use evidence and the experience of caring for patients to lobby for policy change
- Access and shape the changing political landscape
- Build coalitions that increase the pressure for action.

It does this by assisting you to

- Develop and sustain your political leadership ability with the support of a political mentor and coach
- Use a 'live' policy issue to have direct policy impact
- Develop and action strategies to shape policy goals
- Communicate clear messages to gain the support of stakeholders
- Lobby effectively
- Gain direct access to policymakers, politicians, assemblies and parliaments
- Engage successfully with the media
- Identify and work with a constituency of support and build coalitions that work
- Understand the workings of government
- Clarify how ministers and civil servants draw up health and social policy

---

The programme is unique in its design and uses specially developed tools such as the Political Leadership in Action model (Antrobus 2002), shown in Figure 5.1. This 11-step model of influence has been developed inductively from the accounts of nurses who have successfully shaped government policy.

Figure 5.2 depicts the three core elements of the programme:

- Applying political theory to real 'life' policy issues
- Learning experientially about the political process by developing a proposal for policy change on an issue of importance to patients, nurses or nursing using the Political Leadership in Action model

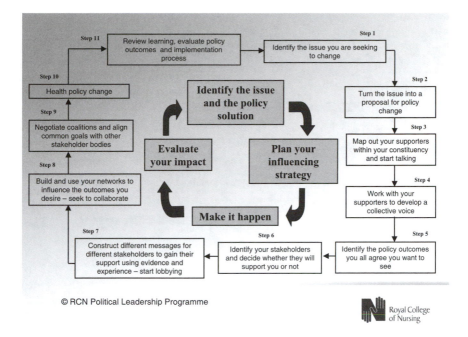

© RCN Political Leadership Programme

Royal College
of Nursing

Figure 5.1 Political Leadership in Action: influencing policymaking

● Documenting the personal development experienced.

Facilitated action learning sets (Revans 1980) integrate these three core elements and provide peer support and challenge. Participants use a specially designed political leadership self-assessment tool and personal development plan to measure their personal progress. A structured portfolio has also been developed for participants to use to document their learning and collate evidence of the impact and engagement they are having in the policymaking arena.

Evaluation: methods

The type of approach used in an evaluation should reflect the focus and context of the evaluation. Øvretveit (1999) distinguishes between four evaluation approaches, experimental, managerial, developmental and economic. The developmental approach is considered to be a flexible formative approach with close continual links between the findings and subsequent action to be taken. Parlett (1981) describes the key features of this approach as follows:

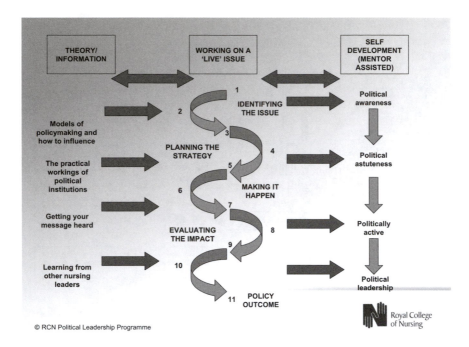

Figure 5.2 The RCN's Political Leadership Programme

The basic emphasis of this approach is on interpreting, in each study, a variety of educational practices, participants' experiences, institutional procedures and management problems in ways that are useful and recognisable to those for whom the study is made.

(Parlett 1981)

The 'macro' domain (Antrobus 2003) or political context in which evaluating the impact of political leadership development is to take place is a difficult concept to define given the dynamic factors that influence it, such as the particular ambitions of the nurses in question, national and local politics, organizational characteristics, relationships, perceived barriers and culture. These contextual factors are challenges explored more fully in baseline assessments carried out prior to delivery of the political leadership programme to any given cohort of participants. A developmental approach therefore is arguably the most appropriate and relevant evaluation approach in which to evaluate the impact of political leadership development for nurses.

Within a developmental evaluation framework several evaluators have noted the relevance of pragmatic evaluation (Chelimsky 1997; Scriven 1997). A pragmatic evaluation, as suggested by its name, rejects methodological purism (Shaw 1999) in favour of using pluralistic methods in order to understand an intervention in a complex social context where outcomes are difficult to predict, but require to be evaluated within the confines of a project timetable. The nature of a pragmatic evaluation, as in most developmental evaluations, implies some degree of participation from the programme participants. In a critical review of approaches to participation in evaluation theory, Gregory (2000) concludes that the nature and effectiveness of participation, whichever approach is chosen, is a problematic and neglected area of evaluation theory research. Therefore it should be borne in mind that the impact of the programme on delegates participating in the programme evaluation is not fully understood and some degree of trade off between relevance and rigour can be expected. However, the RCN political leadership project team consider that participation and ownership of the evaluation by the programme participants is important in order to inform the processes and outcomes in striving for greater lobbying capability. While Hammersley (1995) opposed pragmatic evaluation in terms of the validity of the evaluation, the RCN PLP team concur with the views of Taket and White (1997), who considered that evaluation is a social process that is focused around the needs of the participants and not purely scientific in order that the end results are meaningful and relevant. Therefore, the evaluations to date incorporated in the RCN PLP have adopted a developmental, pragmatic approach using pluralistic data collection methods to best capture the complex, unpredictable and culturally different social context in which our nurses are working both nationally and internationally.

Antrobus et al. (2004) describe a four-stage journey of political leadership development as the participant's progress through the programme which offers a useful evaluation framework when exploring acquisition of political leadership skills. The four stages are outlined in Table 5.1.

Table 5.1 Four stages of political leadership development

STAGE OF POLITICAL LEADERSHIP DEVELOPMENT	DESCRIPTOR
Political awareness	Developing an understanding of how to get things done in an organization and of how power is distributed.
Political astuteness	Work beyond the boundaries of my own work, actively influencing the local health system and being able to analyse situations and engage with others in a 'politically intelligent way'.

| Politically active | Interact and network with the wider health and social care community, including politicians and policymakers on issues of concern. |
| Political leadership | Involved in policy communities, actively lobby to bring about policychange and compile evidence on my own impact on the policy making processes. |

Source: Antrobus et al. (2004)

Table 5.1 describes the progression that Antrobus et al. (2004) observe as programme participants develop their political leadership skills, working through the 11-step model.

The programme portfolios offer units of analyses for single case study evaluation (Yin 2003) and have been used to illustrate the extent to which programme participants have engaged in the policymaking arena (Antrobus et al. 2005). Yin (2003) describes how the format of presenting case studies can be a narrative, that is participants' portfolio of evidence. As the portfolios are lengthy, Yin (2003) suggests that data are presented in response to a question or series of questions. The programme evaluation therefore has reported summaries of the portfolios submitted at the end of the programme in response to the single question.

'Has the participant progressed in the policymaking arena?'

The detailed 11-step model (described in Figure 5.1) underpinning progression through the programme provides definitions against which outcomes in the political arena by the programme participants can be evaluated. Self-assessment of personal and political leadership development is elicited through an evaluation proforma completed on the final programme day which includes a self-assessment of political leadership capability, using the four descriptors of political leadership development described in Table 5.1. Data concerning individual learning, assessment of progression of policy goals, support given by coaches and mentors and plans for ongoing political work are also gathered through the proforma and can be thematically analysed (Morse and Field 1995).

To illustrate the political leadership development that participants undergo, evaluation data from the 2005 political leadership programme are described. Following delivery of the programme in 2005, 15 portfolios, one combined from two participants, were submitted for analysis representing 62 per cent response rate from the whole cohort. The portfolios of evidence submitted were summarized in response to the question 'Has the participant progressed in the policymaking arena?' Ten case studies are given here that describe participants' journeys through the 11-step model in a variety of different political contexts.

Case study 5.1 Helping practice nurses to have a greater knowledge of the children's National Service Framework (NSF) through professional development

Polly generated a comprehensive stakeholder map including RCN primary care and practice nursing representatives, editors of relevant journals, a Strategic Health Authority lead nurse, a higher education representative and RCN regional boards. Polly used her mentor and political coach to facilitate contact with these stakeholders. Polly developed an influencing strategy grounded in policy documents and stories relevant to patient care and maintained contact with the stakeholders throughout the programme. Polly published an article in the *Nursing Times*, which led to a subsequent invitation to write a book chapter. In her role within the RCN Institute, Polly pursued her policy goal through RCN channels of communication such as the learning zone and congress.

Case study 5.2 Supporting learning disability nurses to ensure their continued recognition as nurses through organizational changes

Robert used the programme planning tool to identify where to start pursuing his goal. Reflecting on the complexity of political lobbying and the need to form coalitions, the policy goal was further refined. Robert met with national stakeholders including the chairman of independent sector 'modernizing nursing careers', Stephen Rose, chief executive of Choice Support, who facilitated a meeting for Robert to meet with the Chief Nursing Officer, Christine Beasley, to raise awareness of these issues. Robert also raised awareness with the Director of Mental Health Nursing at the Department of Health and with NHS employers. He formed a 'supporting nurses through change' reference group and worked with the RCN centrally and in his local branch, which culminated in the submission of an RCN resolution.

Case study 5.3 Enhancing the profile of older people's nursing by developing and promoting positive images

Clare's policy work followed on from the work of a previous political leadership programme participant from her forum. Clare detailed her objectives in relation to her policy goal both within and externally to the RCN, for example by contributing to existing work within the RCN, through RCN publications and at congress. Externally, Clare linked with the Department of Health Older People's Nurse, who following a meeting came to visit Clare in her clinical area. Clare has raised awareness and pursued her policy goals in a number of arenas for example by developing a 'marketing' angle to a student nurse toolkit, contributing to a regional event and producing an article 'Why chose to work with older people?'.

Case study 5.4 Offering alternatives to adults with tuberculosis (TB) unable to complete their prescribed course of treatment

During the programme Malcolm mapped stakeholders while simultaneously identifying benefits and non-benefits for each of being offered admission to an appropriate care setting until they have completed their treatment. Working with the RCN communications team, Malcolm was invited to join the All Party Parliamentary Advisory Group on Global TB. Working with specialist colleagues, Malcolm was able to produce a policy document for the group's consideration, although this was ultimately rejected.

Case Study 5.5 Considering and influencing the policy and guidelines offered by the RCN in respect of the issue of self-harm

Ian prepared abstracts grounded in evidence for 'safe cutting' and published these on the RCN website prior to congress where the issue was debated. Awareness raising included a front page article in the *Sunday Times*, and a RCN Women's Mental Health Group workshop and RCN prison nursing forum conference. The conference was jointly hosted by the RCN and NHS Scotland forensic mental health services managed care networks. This national conference was used to distribute a questionnaire to accumulate more evidence and disseminate the experiences of patients who self-harm. Throughout the programme Ian facilitated discussion and raised awareness on the RCN discussion zone about the issue.

Case study 5.6 Influencing government departments to agree to use the same criteria and definitions as part of a single assessment process

Liz developed a detailed project plan and body of evidence (which included talking to stakeholders, e.g. patients, disabled rights officer and GPs). To enable children and adults who have disability, which may be physical, cognitive or learning disability or a combination to access services or benefits in a more cost effective and efficient manner. Uniform definitions and criteria would improve prevalence data. She assessed the extra workload created for GPs by not having a single assessment process and built this into her body of evidence. During the programme Liz documented continuing stakeholder engagement, for example with the chief executive of the Spinal Injuries Association, policy officials at the Department of Health and engaged the help of her MP, who worked with Liz to prepare a parliamentary question, which opened up a further opportunity for a supplementary question. Liz raised awareness through submission of an article to a nursing journal and widely distributing a briefing paper to key political stakeholders, for example the Care Services Minister in the House of Commons.

Case study 5.7 Developing and implementing infection control guidelines for the post-operative recovery area

Gillian compiled a comprehensive action plan to pursue her policy issue. She formed a guideline working group within her forum steering group, which following a literature search produced a policy guideline by the end of the programme. While drafting the guideline, Gillian raised awareness through the forum newsletter, local RCN branch, the RCN website, a fringe event at the 2006 RCN congress and used the latter opportunity to gather more evidence through a questionnaire distributed to participants. She worked with her political coach who had previously been successful in the related RCN 'Wipe it out' campaign and was keen to support the development of the guideline. Gillian formed coalitions with the Infection Control Nurses Association and the RCN infection control adviser. She documented plans to consult with and have the guidelines ratified by the four UK chief nursing officers in Spring 2007 and other associated national nursing groups and affiliated organizations, e.g. the National Patient Safety Organization and the RCN Institute Gillian documented her intention to present the guideline at the 2007 forum conference and have an official launch following the consultation. Gillian took over as chair of her forum during the course of the programme.

Case study 5.8 Pursuing a recognized qualification for nurses in aesthetic medicine

With the proposed regulation of cosmetic surgery, the emphasis on quality care and the protection of the public, the time is right for there to be a recognized qualification for nurses in aesthetic medicine. Elizabeth gathered the need for the qualification (postgraduate diploma) by surveying members of the Aesthetic Nurses' Forum. She published her findings in the forum newsletter and in an associated journal stating that the majority of nurses working in the field supported this development, were willing to undertake further training and ongoing continuous professional development. Throughout the programme Elizabeth documented the usefulness in the programme tools, e.g. benefits realization exercise and documented support in the learning set, both during the programme and at congress, to pursue her goals. On completion of the programme Elizabeth identified the next steps needed to secure sponsorship for the programme as well as support from the Nursing and Midwifery Council and Healthcare commission. The programme is now established in institutes of higher education.

Case study 5.9 Ensuring user involvement in the development of the evidence base for nursing

Tracey created a detailed action plan with timescales at the start of the programme and approached the Director of Patient Experience and Public Involvement at the National Patient Safety Agency to be her political mentor. Rallying support through existing networks, letters and emails, she formed a national advisory group, consisting of representatives from higher education, RCN forums, voluntary sector organizations, clinical practice to create RCN guidelines meeting her policy goal. Tracey engaged with the RCN both at regional board and in the RCN Institute which led to her policy issue being part of the 2006 RCN core business agenda. Tracey raised awareness in the nursing press by publishing editorials and letters. Wishing to influence fundholders to promote user involvement in research, during the course of the programme, Tracey was invited to join the UKCRC Patient and Public involvement group which has an influential voice with commissioners. Having spearheaded the publication of RCN guidance documents she continued working with the RCN marketing department to raise awareness for RCN members through flyers, web-based information, dedicated workshops and a planned launch of the guidelines at the RCN research conference 2007.

Case Study 10 Establishing national guidelines for the requesting of X-rays by nurses and other non-medical health care practitioners, endorsed by relevant professional bodies

Jenny progressed her policy goal with support from the programme, her political mentor and coach. She gathered evidence, ensuring her goal was aligned with existing national policy, to support her political goal. Jenny identified her stakeholders and formed coalitions with professional bodies and within the RCN both through her local board and centrally. This included the Society of Radiographers, Chartered Society of Physiotherapists, British School of Osteopathy, NHS Alliance and Department of Health. Continuing to raise awareness through professional journals, newsletters and seminars and keeping abreast of press coverage, Jenny worked with colleagues and published an RCN guideline supporting her goal in November 2006. A communication strategy to raise awareness of the publication was created resulting in press releases in nursing journals, web-based information and communication with strategic health authorities, primary care trusts and all four UK chief nursing officers. Jenny ensured evaluation of the guidelines can take place through anecdotal evidence, surveys, and hits on the RCN website and through RCN direct.

Personal development

Participants were asked to reflect on their political leadership capability at the start and at the end of the programme. At the start of the programme, three of the fourteen participants described themselves as both politically aware and active, two participants described themselves as politically aware, active and leading. At the end of the programme seven participants described themselves as politically astute, active and leading and two participants described themselves as operating in all four categories. Overall there was a clear shift from participants being political aware/astute at the start of the programme to being politically astute, active and leading by the end of the programme. This transition is described from the perspective of the following participant:

> "I can identify the difference between the start and the end as being more focused and surer of my facts. These facts have been questioned, refined and redeveloped and has allowed me to be more assertive when challenging. These skills have been developed not only through the PLP but through other activities such as the lobbying, working together and everyday representation."

Reflecting on the nature of developing political leadership skills several participants commented on the strategic nature of political leadership and the need to be clear about whom to influence. The following quote is illustrative:

> "That it [political leadership] is very strategic and not for the fainthearted. That much of it is about networks and positions of influence and developing a high profile in your field/policy issue before."

Similarly another participant describes how the programme helped to give more detailed insight into this process: 'The PLP showed me a deeper way of analyzing problems and getting to the central core'.

By the end of the programme several participants also reflected on their own achievements and realized that they could be in a position of influence:

> "I can do it [politically lead]. I have most of the skills. It takes a lot of persistence, you have to hold people to deadlines and you need time to get the right people."

Learning the skills of lobbying was also a common theme in participants learning and personal development from the programme, as the following quotation describes:

> "It [lobbying] does not have to be confrontational or involve marches etc. Some objectives can be met by influencing behind the scenes. Issues are not time limited but continue beyond the PLP. I have learned so much about media, networking, influencing, leadership, systems of government, the Department of Health."

Reflections like these described are evident in all the evaluations of the programme to date.

The transferability of the 12-month programme in an international context is borne out by participants documenting success in the Malopolska region in Poland. The following quotation from Dr Maria Kozka, county consultant for nursing affairs, describes the group's success 12 months after the group refined its political goal to legally regulate nursing standards in nursing homes:

> "Currently myself and Tadek [Chair of Malapolska chambers] co-ordinate the nurses who work in nursing homes – and we now have the representation that we wanted. As of now the county sheriff's offices send out all parliamentary papers to myself, the Chambers and Union for consultation. We have demonstrated that nursing is an independent profession governed by our own abided laws. We had lengthy discussions with a member of parliament and said that nurses need to be educated. In the meeting it is not just one individual who is appointed by the group to go

but it's a whole group effort. So we have managed to take over the management of long-term care in nursing homes."

Additionally, over the period of programme delivery the membership of the Polish Nursing Association (PNA) had increased by 80 per cent in the Krakow region. There were 100 new registered PNA members, new branches and new interest groups. Participants reported that the profile of nursing appeared to have been raised regionally and nationally by using the media in the form of radio and television panels. Eleven newspaper and journal articles were published in the final six months of programme delivery. Academic links were used to promote the concept of political leadership and the group's project work through nurse education, chambers publications and academic journals.

As outlined earlier in the chapter there has been little evidence found in the international literature of the impact of political leadership programmes specifically designed for nurses. While the evaluation does have limitations, the findings raise some interesting questions in the following three areas:

- Improving nurses' engagement with policymakers and politicians
- The future design of political leadership programmes
- The role of NNAs in the development of nursing as a collective lobbying force.

Each of these areas will be discussed in turn.

Improving nurses' engagement with policymakers and politicians

For those nurses who wish to develop their political skills, a political leadership programme designed within and accessed through a NNA can prove useful. Actioning 'live' policy issues provides an important experiential component to leadership development. This enables nurses to learn while they are actually doing policy work. Being coached, while engaging politically, would appear to increase nurses' confidence, an essential prerequisite in any kind of leadership development.

Members lobbying through a PLP, on behalf of a NNA, is not without its risks, however. Crucial to effective political action is consistency of message and a collective lobbying voice. The challenge for participants, political coaches and the programme team is to ensure that there is a constituency of wider membership and organizational support for the policy goals that are being lobbied for.

The personal development framework offered for consideration within this chapter, while rudimentary, does offer some valuable insights into the journey that nurses undertake to develop themselves as political leaders. Subsequent evaluations could usefully explore the framework further. While there was some evidence that nurses became politically active in the way that they had begun to engage with the political process and politicians and policymakers, evidence of political leadership through directly shaping policy is still in its early development.

Policymaking is, however, subject to the vagaries of the political process and participants could be extremely skilled within the political arena but the timing of their policy issue means that their policy impact may be minimal. Waiting for opportunities for policy change, which may not happen over the 12 months of the programme may mean that the evaluation should be developed on a longitudinal basis over time.

The future design of political leadership programmes

There are many positive comments on the impact of the programme overall from both participants and stakeholders. Future evaluations should pay more attention to the tools and interventions used to understand exactly what impact each has on the personal development journey of participants.

Learning about *how* to develop nurses for political leadership has been the prime achievement of the programme. This knowledge, currently held by the programme team, could be disseminated further in a toolkit for facilitators so that the programme design can be reproduced within other NNAs internationally.

The self-assessment tool used by participants is still being validated and its reliability as a political leadership assessment tool for nurses' needs to be developed. More work also needs to be done to refine the PL in action model in order to develop its usefulness further within other contexts.

The role of NNAs in the development of nursing as a collective lobbying force

While much has been made of nursing leadership in the international literature, little has been made of the role of NNAs in relation to leadership development. We argue that NNAs can play a crucial role in developing nursing as a collective lobbying force and in co-ordinating effort around key policy priorities. NNAs can build and sustain a network of Political Leaderships (PLs) in nursing who have been through a PLP and are then able to actively work on campaigns and national election activities.

This does require investment however by the NNA on behalf of its members. Nurses need to understand *how* to engage politically. NNAs also need to build a body of evidence of effective political action in order to consider the most productive way to improve their lobbying capability. The results of investment in PL development and the underpinning research then needs to be disseminated on an international basis.

Conclusion

Despite calls since the early 1980s for nurses to get more political, there are few countries internationally where nurses and nursing issues can be seen to have had a significant impact on the local or national policy agendas.

The evaluation reported here demonstrates the positive impact that PLPs run through a NNA can have. Nurses on the programme:

- Gain confidence in their ability to network and lobby and influence politicians and policymakers
- Develop a more sophisticated understanding of how policy is influenced and how political institutions work
- Increase the impact of the policy and political activity within their specialist area of expertise
- Describe a personal development journey and their transformation towards political leadership.

If NNAs are to influence health and social policy it would seem reasonable to suggest that investing in PLPs could pay useful dividends. Creating an international 'political leadership network' of NNAs could strengthen the 'political intelligence' and evidence base nurses need to shape policies and importantly make a real difference to patients and communities on health issues locally, nationally and globally.

Key points

- Nurses potentially have a vital role to play in shaping health policies.
- There is limited knowledge about how to prepare nurses to influence policy effectively and limited understanding of the skills and knowledge needed for effective political leadership.
- Detailed description is offered on how to prepare nurses to contribute effectively to policymaking processes.
- The role of national nursing associations in political leadership is examined.

Reflective exercises

1 How successful are national nursing associations in driving the nursing policymaking agenda?

2 What skills are required for nurses to be politically effective both individually and collectively?

3 How might you assess the success of any political leadership activity in nursing?

4 What links do you have with any political or national forum?

5 If you were to devise an action plan as described in the case studies, what key issue would you highlight, and who would you want to lobby?

References

Antrobus, S. (2002) *Strategic Guidelines for Influencing Health Policy*. London: Royal College of Nursing.

Antrobus, S. (2003) What is political leadership? *Nursing Standard* 17(43): 40–44.

Antrobus, S. (2004) Why does nursing need political leaders? *Journal of Nursing Management* 12(4): 227–228.

Antrobus, S. and Kitson, A. (1999) Nursing leadership: influencing and shaping health policy and nursing practice. *Journal of Advanced Nursing* 29(3): 746–753.

Antrobus, S., Macleod, A. and Bailey, J. (2004) Scaling the political ladder. *Nursing Management* 11(7): 23–28.

Antrobus, S., Macleod, A. and Bailey, J. (2005) *RCN Forum Political Leadership Programme Evaluation 2005*, RCN Reports (unpublished). London: Royal College of Nursing.

Bell, D.S., Hargrove, E.C. and Theakston, K. (1999) Skill in context: a comparison of politicians. *Presidential Studies Quarterly* 29(3): 528–548.

Buerhaus, P. (1992) Teaching health care public policy. *Nursing and Health Care* 13(6): 304–309.

Canadian Nurses Association (2000) Nursing is a political act – the bigger picture. *Nursing Now* 8.

Chelimsky, E. (1997) Thoughts for a new Evaluation Society. *Evaluation* 1(1): 97–104.

Cohen, S., Mason, D., Kovner, C., Leavitt, J., Pulcinin, J. and Sochalski, J. (1996) Stages of nursing's political development: where we've been and where we ought to go. *Nursing Outlook* 44: 259–266.

Cunningham, G. and Kitson, A. (2000) An evaluation of the RCN clinical leadership programme, Part 1 and Part 2. *Nursing Standard* 15(12): 34–37 and 15(13): 34–40.

Ehlers, V.J. (2000) Nursing and politics: a South African perspective. *International Nursing Review* 47: 74–82.

Game, C. (1979) Review essay: on local political leadership. *Policy and Politics* 7(4): 395–408.

Gregory, A. (2000) Problematizing participation: a critical review of approaches to participation in evaluation theory. *Evaluation* 6(2): 179–199.

Hambleton, R. (1998) Strengthening political leadership in UK local government. *Public Money and Management* 18(1): 41–52.

Hammersley, M. (1995) *The Politics of Social Research*. London: Sage.

Hennessy, D. (2000) The emerging themes. In D. Hennessy and P. Spurgeon (eds) *Health Policy and Nursing: Influence, Development and Impact*. London: Macmillan.

International Council of Nurses (ICN) (2002) *Impact and Sustainability of the Leadership for Change Project*. Geneva: ICN.

Kotter, J. and Lawrence, P. (1974) *Mayors in Action: Five Approaches to Urban Governance*. New York: Wiley.

Leach, S. and Wilson, D. (2002) Rethinking local political leadership. *Public Administration* 80(4): 665–689.

Maslin-Prothero, S. and Masterson, A. (2002) Power, politics and nursing in the United Kingdom. *Policy, Politics & Nursing Practice* 3(2): 108–117.

Mason, D.J., Leavitt, J.K. and Chaffee, M.W. (2002) Policy and politics: a framework for action. In D.J. Mason, J.K. Leavitt and M.W. Chaffee *Policy and Politics in Nursing and Health Care*, 4th edn. St Louis, MO: Saunders (Elsevier Science).

Masterson, A. and Maslin-Prothero, S. (eds) (1999) *Nursing and Politics: Power through Practice*. Edinburgh: Churchill Livingstone.

Morse, J.M. and Field, P.A. (1995) *Qualitative Research Methods for Health Professionals*, 2nd edn. London: Sage.

Øvretveit, J. (1999) *Evaluating Health Interventions*. Buckingham: Open University Press.

Parlett, M. (1981) Illuminative evaluation. In J. Øvretveit (1999) *Evaluating Health Interventions*. Buckingham: Open University Press.

Rafferty, A-M. (1995) *Political Leadership in Nursing: The Role of Nursing in Health Care Reform*. Final Harkness Fellowship Report (unpublished).

Revans, R. (1980) What is action learning? *Journal of Management Development* 1(3): 64–75.

Scriven, M. (1997) Truth and objectivity in evaluation. In E. Chelimsky and W. Shadish (eds) *Evaluation for the 21st Century*. Thousand Oaks, CA: Sage.

Shaw, I.F. (1999) *Qualitative Evaluation*. London: Sage.

Siegel, M.E. (2001) Lessons in leadership from three American Presidents. *Journal of Leadership Studies* 8(1): 34–47.

Taket, A. and White, l. (1997) Working with heterogeneity: a pluralist strategy for evaluation. *Systems Research and Behavioural Science* 14(2): 101–111.

Taylor, G. (1995) Politics and nursing: an elective experience. *Journal of Advanced Nursing* 21(3): 1180–1185.

West, E. and Scott, C. (2000) Nursing in the public sphere: breaking the boundaries between research and policy. *Journal of Advanced Nursing* 32(4): 817–824.

Woolnough, H. and Faugier, J. (2002) An evaluative study assessing the impact of the Leading an Empowered Organisation (LEO) programme. *Journal of Research in Nursing* 7(6): 412–427.

Yin, R.K. (2003) *Case Study Research: Design and Methods*, 3rd edn. London: Sage.

6 Educating leaders for global health care

Dawn Freshwater, Iain Graham and Philip Esterhuizen

Overview

In this chapter we discuss how the provision of nursing care, and the role of nursing in the multidisciplinary health care team, has never been more complex, and the demands on health care professionals to forge multi-professional, multidisciplinary and inter-agency partnerships in the provision of that care are great. Constant technological and medical advances, coupled with an ever-increasing and ageing population with constantly raised expectations, have a knock-on effect on staffing levels, nurses' and AHPs' responsibilities and on the health care workforce overall. This impacts in both a positive and a negative manner. The scope for health care professionals to enjoy a breadth of areas in which to work, and paradoxically the possibility for burnout and reduction in standards of care is unprecedented. Leadership, as never before, is a fundamental challenge to health care professionals. Underlining this challenge is the need for educational institutions and educationalists to provide a framework for the development and support of future health care leaders.

Introduction

We are basing this chapter on the premise that the development of leadership and the knowledge that underpins nursing and therapists' leadership – indeed defines it – must also be established as part of a community of knowledge building. There are numerous leadership programmes in existence which attempt to promote leadership abilities and skills in order to maintain, co-ordinate and improve the provision of health care as it currently stands and therefore of nursing. An excellent example is described in Chapter 5 by Antrobus and colleagues. We do not argue against these programmes; they are necessary and should be better subscribed to. However, the world is changing at such a fast pace and what is needed are health care leaders who can navigate and travel new frontiers, provide visions that will engage health professionals, for the benefit of quality health care provision.

If nurses and others are to maximize their role and be crucial participants in the future development and design of health care, then educational institutions across the world have a responsibility to prepare them for international leadership positions.

In this chapter we focus on the role of educational programmes to support and facilitate the development of effective and transformational leaders. We explore the impact of health care changes globally and their effects on health care professionals, in particular on nurses. These dynamics have major implications for the development and nurturing of nurse leaders of the future. In considering an educational strategy to support future leaders we also briefly examine the significance of doctoral education and the role of mentorship and coaching.

As mentioned elsewhere in this book, nursing is changing almost as rapidly as the context in which it is practised. As a dynamic profession, nursing is responsive and is adapting to meet the needs of both patients and the public and indeed its key stakeholders. Across the globe, nurses have taken on new roles, work across boundaries, and are setting up new services to meet patients' needs. Similarly AHPs are doing likewise, as is evidenced in Chapter 4. So it is timely then to draw breath at this point and in doing so, consider what these changes imply for leadership in health care, and to work towards ensuring that in the future health care is led efficiently, productively and with conscious purpose. Importantly health care requires leadership that can move people as well as organizations to transform and advance nursing and AHPs in the global context. The challenge for educationalists is to find creative ways in which they can support leaders to develop those skills required in a global economy of health, while simultaneously transforming the profession.

The changing nature of health care

It is without question that modern health services across Western societies are undergoing unprecedented reform and change. Health care systems are and will continue to face major global and societal changes. A number of factors lie behind government policies to reform the way the health service works, including:

- Society today is more complex, giving rise to greater social, cultural, racial and geographical diversity.
- There are more people in the older age range so long-term conditions are more prevalent. As a consequence demand for health and social care will continue to rise.
- Major causes of morbidity and mortality such as heart disease and some cancers can respond well to preventative measures, but these frequently require lifestyle changes which can be hard to achieve.
- Health is not distributed equally and inequalities continue to be a major challenge.
- The working population is smaller so fewer people are available to enter the profession.
- People's expectations of health care are changing. They are more knowledgeable and expect to be treated as partners and equals, and to have choices and option available to them.
- Rapid advances in technology mean more effective treatments as well as the ability to provide care in different settings.
- The cost of new treatments and new information and communication technologies means a greater focus on value for money.

Current reform programmes seem to feature the following main characteristics:

- Putting the needs and preferences of patients, users and the public, rather than those of professionals, at the forefront of decisions about patterns of services
- Focusing on integrated care based on individualized pathways across local health economies and social care
- Enabling much more choice for individuals
- Improving the care of people with long-term conditions
- Placing greater emphasis on prevention, health promotion and supporting self-care
- Moving more care outside of acute hospitals into the community and people's homes
- Providing incentives for working in new ways.

As the health professionals who usually provide constant care, the success of these health care reforms depends heavily on the contribution of nurses: they are, alongside other health care professionals, responsible for delivering the care that patients want. Nurses know that if they are to meet patients' needs in a variety of care settings, the values of their profession must remain. Wherever nurses work, there are four elements to the nurse's role that straddle geographical and disciplinary boundaries:

- Practice
- Education, training and development
- Quality and service development
- Leadership, management and supervision.

Nurses will continue to care for people who cannot care for themselves, will support and empower people with long-term health care problems to care for themselves, and help people to promote their own health. This will apply to children, young people, adults and older people. The role of the nurses in carrying out these roles and responsibilities will, however, continue to change in line with the health reforms that are improving care for patients. An aspect of change that should be taken into account when considering health reforms is that they appear to focus largely on output and production, linked to risk reduction, rather than quality of care related to the art of caring. Neither is there specific mention of nurses' role in supporting a peaceful death. Palliative care, for example, often appears to be assigned as a specialist area rather than being integrated as a generic role specific to the nursing domain. As such changes are defined, refined and redefined, the nursing workforce will need to:

- Organize care around the needs of patients and clients, including end-of-life care.
- Ensure patients have a good experience of nursing as reputations of organizations and patient choice will rest on the quality of nursing.
- Work in a range of settings, crossing hospital and community care, and use telemedicine.
- Have the skills and competencies to care for older people, and people with long-term conditions, which may have both physical and mental health needs.
- Be able to use preventative and health promotion interventions.
- Work for diverse employers, and take opportunities for self-employment where appropriate.
- Have sufficient numbers of nurses with advanced level skills to meet demand.
- Work as leaders and members of multidisciplinary teams inside and outside hospital, and across health and social care teams.
- Work with new forms of practitioners, for example assistant practitioners and anaesthesia practitioners.
- Deliver high productivity and best value for money.

It could be argued then that given this dynamic context, which will shape the emerging leadership of the nursing profession, there are certain key issues that need to be considered for those institutions and educationalists involved in directing training and development programmes. A careful integration of all four elements of nursing can, in our view, be used as a platform for advancing the maturity of profession through leading by *expertise* rather than purely from *experience*.

Changing roles and leadership skills

The first point that we wish to dwell on here relates to the position of nurses in a team of health professionals both established and new. Relationships with physicians may become fraught as turf battles break out (see Chapter 3) and governments, through legislation, empower nurses to have prescription rights, diagnostics access and resource allocation. A current issue for many Westernized countries, determining who does what and how new types of health practitioner will be accommodated, requires leadership solutions. Importantly, it should not be forgotten that the role of the patient or client and their significant other will also change. Not only are they dealing with issues of empowerment, but also there is an expectation that individuals will do more with regard to their health status. This change in the demands and expectations of an individual patient and their carer extends to the debate on choices related to end-of-life discussion and decisions.

An important aspect of forward thinking leadership is to address these – often philosophical – discussions with staff ahead of time. The increase in requests for assisted death is becoming increasingly apparent as the media exposes society and health care professionals to legal and moral battles, fought in the public arena, highlighting the individual's right to choose. Although not all health professionals will be happy with this development and may feel unable to support development in this direction, there is the issue of nurses traditionally being seen as the patient's advocate. A particular challenge for leaders in the development of health care professions, and nursing in particular – if nurses are to retain a pivotal role in health care – will be to embrace the moral imperatives occurring in society. A society which, in our view, is becoming more liberal and reinterpreting traditional Western norms and values, while at the same time embracing new citizens from other cultures and needing to integrate seemingly conservative mores. Leadership skills will be required not only in terms of such independent enablement but also with regard to providing a vision and guidance to accommodate such change for colleagues and peers.

The manner by which nurses meet their accountability to the society they serve also determines a degree of leadership skills. We would argue that curriculum, pedagogy, assessment registration licensure and certification is no longer fit for purpose, steeped as it is in a nineteenth-century model. One could suggest that a convergence into a unified approach to monitoring and evaluating the competence, capability and capacity of nurses and nursing will emerge. Skills passports, which bring together various tools and frameworks to detail essential knowledge and skills required by health care professionals (see for example Skills for Health 2007) are fundamental to advanced education programmes. They focus not only on advanced skills but also on the process of learning how to learn, thereby facilitating far reaching transfer of skills and knowledge across contexts, boundaries and levels of care.

In many instances this is either already instituted or in development as nurses are expected to maintain portfolios of learning activities and achievements (see Jasper 1995; Trossman 1999; LCVV 2001; Rolfe et al. 2001). These portfolios are, however, largely clinically oriented and are often seen as a means of control by the registering professional bodies, rather than the individual practitioner seeing this activity as their personal passport to developing knowledge and (transferable) skills. Herein lies a specific challenge for future leaders. Such an initiative demands that nursing and its underpinning educational philosophy is challenged to address entry to practice based on educational preparation and the ability to deal with the issues generated by the definition of specialism, advanced and generalized practice. Leaders in health care need to subscribe to maintaining their own portfolio development in order to understand and develop insight into their personal development. Although the principles of decision making and critical thinking are transferable between clinical and leadership, the situations can, simultaneously, be very different. This, we believe, necessitates the development and support of leaders who can consider these issues and develop solutions so that the globalization of the workforce in health care can maximize its potential and capitalize on its assets, namely its young talent and committed and determined experts.

Education for leadership

Gender and socialization

Chapter 2 describes the relationship between leadership and management in detail and as such we will not journey any further into that area. However, we are interested in certain qualities that can be described as pertaining to both the ability to lead and the capacity to manage. Kim et al. (2006) argue that effective leaders bring sustainable results, and that in finding their own voice, they inspire others to find theirs. Numbering more than 11 million around the world, nurses constitute the largest number of health care providers in the health care system. While the profession continues to be a female-dominated profession, until just over a decade ago, women held a minority of nursing management positions and very few senior management positions (Alimo-Metcalfe 1993, 1995). The discussion around gender stereotypes has made way for dialogue suggesting that effective leadership requires a balance of male and female qualities; these include strong, assertive, powerful and nurturing, emotional and inclusive qualities (James 1998; Yoder 2001; Kim et al. 2006). Kim et al. (2006) note that women who exhibit characteristics associated with the male traits are perceived as being cold and demanding. Those who invest in others are seen as weak (Mavin 2006). This indicates the importance of significant and consistent mentorship in the development of emotional intelligence, which we believe is pivotal to the development of an effective but individual leadership style (Herbert and Edgar 2004; Cummings et al. 2005; Walsh 2007).

Emotional intelligence (EI) is closely aligned with emotional literacy and can be described as being about a set of non-cognitive abilities that influence the individual's capacity to succeed in life (Stickley and Freshwater 2002). EI works in collaboration with IQ to enhance overall performance, however, it is argued that EI can be measured and it can be learned and it is this ability that differentiates exceptional from mediocre ability and achievement and potentially inspirational leadership (Freshwater and Stickley 2004).

The concept of emotional intelligence has been popularized by the authors Daniel Goleman (1995) and Susie Orbach (1994, 1999); however, the term was already well established prior to the work of these well-known contemporary writers. Reuven Bar-On, an Israeli psychologist, developed the first test of emotional intelligence, which has since gained extensive international recognition, having been translated into 15 different languages. More recently Bar-On has developed a 360-degree version of his test and a youth version (Bar-On and Parker 2000). Bar-On's model contains five overall groupings:

- Interpersonal factors
- Intrapersonal factors
- General mood and motivation
- Stress management
- Adaptability.

Goleman's (1995) own model of emotional intelligence includes a range of emotional skills and personality traits, namely self-awareness, self-management, social awareness and social skills. As both of the above models demonstrate emotional literacy is a fundamental component of EI. Issues such as self-awareness, self-management and interpersonal/intrapersonal factors all contribute towards our ability to register our emotional responses.

If the purpose of emotional literacy is to precisely identify and communicate our feelings and inherent in this, our needs, then it follows that emotional literacy is fundamental not just to any caring profession but is an essential element of leadership and indeed effective management. Orbach (1999) and Freshwater and Robertson (2002), in discussing the complexity of emotions, identify a series of stages in the development of emotional literacy. At the simplest level, once an emotion is registered (at all levels of experience) and recognized (or named), it also needs to be queried (pointing us to the complex emotional responses that are embedded within the emotional experience). Moving through these stages allows us to 'rein back aspects of ourselves which we have foisted on others' (Orbach 1999: 3). This has obvious implications for the appropriate development of mature leadership skills and practices.

Emotional maturity is developed not in individual isolation, but through the process of socialization of which learning is an essential part, whether this be as an infant learning from our parents, as a child learning from teachers and peers, or as an adult, learning in the process of becoming a health professional. Nurses, and AHPs in their professional life, clearly work consistently with human emotion, whether this be through pain, discomfort, sadness, relief or hope. Isobel Menzies-Lyth (1970, 1988) spent many years investigating what she called the emotional labour of nursing, identifying the problems that repression and containment of emotions could lead to, not only for the individual, but also for the institution. As such, we contend that emotionally intelligent training programmes are crucial for the development of effective health care leaders. The ability to practice effective leadership while maintaining professional and social boundaries may arguably be the most difficult action that a health care practitioner can execute. As Stickley and Freshwater (2002) note the balancing of the emotional and the rational minds provides a stable platform to develop the art of caring in any therapeutic relationship and fosters the development of personal and professional boundaries, something that is linked to professional accountability, advocacy and emotional responsibility. Surely, key aspects of clinical and professional leadership. Yet, one might question if nurses and other health care professionals are provided with sufficient opportunities for developing emotional intelligence.

From the discussion so far, and the observation of a gender-related discussion to leadership, it can be noted that personal insight and awareness is central to good leadership. According to authors in the area of gender, women in leadership positions gravitate towards democratic and participatory leadership (Kjervik 1979; Park 1996; Kark 2004; Trinidad and Normore 2005) and transformational and inspirational leadership styles (Eagly and Johannesen-Schmidt 2001; Ridgeway 2001). Considering the predominence of women in health care leadership, this should, therefore, result in an embodiment of the objectives aspired to from a transformational perspective. This does not, however, appear to be the case. Farrell (2001) and Freshwater

(2000) discuss the concept of horizontal violence (defined in Freshwater 2000) and abuse within health care. More recently work by Burnes and Pope (2007) has highlighted negative behaviour which may or may not be classified as bullying. This concept of horizontal violence – hostile and aggressive behaviour by individual or group members towards another member or groups – could be strongly associated with how staff are socialized into the health care system at present.

During our searches of global leadership programmes, we observed that specific leadership programmes for women were minimal. While some may feel it to be beneficial to have gender-defined leadership programmes, this approach needs to viewed critically; the alternative argument is that it may not be wise to create an environment in which women are lulled into a false sense of security, only to be confronted with a male-dominated culture outside the confines of the programme. Perhaps more beneficial would be to have open programmes based on the philosophy of transformational leadership with content being related to experiential learning and emotional intelligence; in this way male and female participants would be exposed to dialogue and discussion and, potentially, understand more of each other's logic, thought processes and leadership styles. This approach would need to be facilitated from a reflective perspective and demands expert educational leadership. There are also very few systematic leadership development programmes for senior strategic level nurses; however, in a recent study of top international leaders in nursing who had been in leadership programmes, it was demonstrated that the most influential aspect of that leadership was the role of the mentor (Madison 1994). This role helped to increase confidence, and importantly encouraged the individual to take risks when the situation was appropriate. The most important role of the mentor would be to coach decision making and strategic thought processes when faced with the messiness of everyday practice. Palmer (2006) in her work on fostering leadership through collaboration also emphasizes the influence of effective mentorship, positing that mentorship programmes can pave the way to nursing expertise in governance; assist with putting knowledge into practice; provide support in regard to enhancing abilities and weathering crises. Sherwood and Freshwater (2005) are concerned with such matters. They explored the role of doctoral education in developing nurse leaders arguing that:

> Doctoral education is charged with preparing leaders who can think out of the box and stimulate creative problem solving in others invigorating nurses to claim a voice in crafting a vision of health care delivery that recognizes the essentialness of nursing.
>
> (Sherwood and Freshwater 2005: 58)

While it is important to value academic qualification, it is equally important for the future of nursing leadership to ascertain whether the discussion primarily concerns the (academic) level of education, or whether it is a gender-related discussion needing to be dealt with and perhaps to challenge the current male-dominated discourse. It is an illusion to think that the gender imbalances will change or dissipate within the foreseeable future and so nursing leaders need to identify the challenge and deal with it. The perception of successful women in leadership, previously mentioned, as being 'cold and demanding' and often the lack of support by other women makes the challenge for women in leadership positions even more complex (Mavin 2006). One could suggest that there is a need for women to become aware that they often accept, or buy into, male-dominated systems owing to their current role in society and their socialized gender-related behaviour. Attempting to deconstruct this behaviour could support women in understanding their own position more fully and provide them with strategies to be proactive in addressing the challenges as already have been illustrated.

Workforce and discipline

This gender divide is contextualized by Salvage (2000) in terms of the historical perspectives of the medical-nursing polarization. She goes on to argue the strength of placing the patient centrally in order to focus on the commonality of the two disciplines. This approach is substantiated by an evaluation of schooling on moral decision making targeting all disciplines. It showed that communication and respect improved in departments where medical and nursing staff participated together, whereas the polarization between disciplines became more marked in cases when medical staff chose not to be involved in the schooling programme (Esterhuizen and Kooyman 2001). However positive the initial impact of a cross-discipline appears, all parties should be aware that the current gender debate is anchored in strong historical roots and may require constant attention and development. It concerns not only communication and mutual tolerance, but also the development of a deep understanding and respect of one another's skills, knowledge and expertise, and commitment to a shared vision.

Not only is the gender debate historically defined, but also the composition of the nursing workforce is varied and complex, yet we still hold to a nineteenth-century model of professionalism and definition of a professional. Leadership is needed to challenge these notions and provide views and informed opinion on what professionalism means in the twenty-first century. The concept of leadership needs to be instilled from the start of foundation programmes educating health care staff prior to professional registration. This does not imply managerial skills to run a team, but rather leadership-related thinking skills: critical thinking, self-reflection and emotional intelligence skills. Once newly qualified health care professionals have been socialized into their role within the system, it becomes very difficult to change behaviour. Linked to the workforce debate, the evolution of the new wave of concentration on changing the work environment as a recruitment and retention strategy is propelling nursing beyond the blue-collar syndrome, where nurses were compensated based on an hourly wage. As with other professions that are moving beyond the industrial age, nursing is primed for new leadership strategies, ones that foster transformational changes in education, service delivery, work environments, recruitment and retention, and performance-based compensation.

Traditionally nursing is challenged with the label of being a silent profession. As Sherwood and Freshwater (2005) note:

> Historical developments related to views of nursing as a calling, symbolization as the angel of mercy, socialization derived from being a predominantly female profession, environments entrenched in steep hierarchy, and other societal factors have contributed to the lack of voice attributed to nurses in the decision making arena that drives the health care market.
> (Sherwood and Freshwater 2005: 58)

It is clear that a convergence of many factors, some of which are discussed in this book, offer new opportunities that perhaps are best met with preparation of new leadership skills. A view of nursing that encompasses each nurse as a leader signifies and requires new approaches to leadership development and changes in doctoral curricula. This generation can, with exposure to transformational leaders, help move nursing from silence to voice. Sherwood and Freshwater (2005) perceive doctoral education as making a significant impact on these much needed changes. Global workforce matters suggest the need for health professionals to redefine their roles and purpose, given patient or client requirements for care and technology. All professionals continuously grapple with their identity, their science and their continued research and educational functions. This is highlighted in the current climate and dictates the need for leaders and leadership to help move these crucial agendas of identity and purpose along.

Science and practice

The adoption and development of new science into practice is equally as challenging because in a globalized society with increasing virtual and digital technology, many of the controls and methods once used to test new practices will not be relevant. The development of information systems facilitates faster access to information, coupled with the constant remodelling of the technology. The former dependence on rules, regulations and policies is already being replaced with a strong orientation to the ethical and moral codes of human rights, which in turn will be shaped by the nature of the work that communities of health professionals will create and do. Analysis of treatment outcomes and performance measurement and analysis, already established in the UK will become more firmly entrenched in political and budgetary agendas, linked as they are to health care expenditure and the development of scientific and human resource potential (House of Commons 2000). This will be further highlighted by consumer wishes and expectations, particularly where the consumer exercises choice and desirability. The new-found consumerism in health care will develop still further to incorporate multiple points of entry into the health care system and clients will exercise their rights to remain independent. This shift towards a more market-based health care provision will result in a move away from a medically defined model of care based upon the treatment of pathology to a health and well-being model based perhaps upon the concept on healing centres. Such a development not only breaks with the traditional medical model but also will require a different approach for leadership and perhaps a different preparation for leadership roles.

The way forward: leading the charge

The ramifications of these and of other developments are especially pronounced for nurses because in most countries they represent the largest health care workforce. In order to move forward and ensure a sustainable health care system nurse leaders must address a number of issues which (as we have alluded to) include:

- The profession's diversity and identity
- Multiple points of entry (currently under discussion in the UK)
- Clinical academic career pathways
- Better educational preparation with regard to social, economic and political consideration
- The ageing workforce
- Outdated rules and regimens
- Broader ethical foci
- Changing focus of health care provision.

As with any proposed change, there is little doubt that challenges to professional identity, roles and purpose generate much disruption and anxiety among nurses. Yet such change is simultaneously providing nurses with greater opportunities to develop new and cost-effective models of improving the health and well-being of individuals and their communities.

One of the most important contributions that nurse leaders could make today would be to articulate a coherent vision of the future of both the profession and the health care delivery system. Based on a clear and articulated vision, future nursing leaders need to be able to argue astutely with regard to financial or budgetary restraints, balancing an excellent quality of service provision and staff satisfaction within available funding. Within this discussion they should remain focused on their core values related to staff, their care for patients or clients and their supportive network, without becoming embroiled in economic discussions. In other words, work effectively within a different multidisciplinary context – namely with experts in financial and strategic fields while articulating valid arguments related to quality, efficiency and efficacy. This may entail a proactive approach to develop a set of shared values and visions within the organization and across disciplines and so maintain a dialogue between clinicians and administrators. To do so, leaders will have to adopt four complementary perspectives:

- Focus on core values
- Welcome change as an opportunity to develop the profession and health care, while building on existing skills, knowledge and experience
- Adopt a cosmopolitan outlook to deal with the multiculturalism of society and the plurality of the organization
- Be more able to equate and articulate quality with financial/budgetary restraints.

Nurses' frontline roles in care delivery provide them with intimate knowledge of clinical operations. From this experience, they also gain a number of competencies critical to leadership, including cultural awareness, community focus, conflict management and teamwork skills. However, experience alone is not sufficient to augment the nursing leadership courses taught at the basic level. Nurses require additional leadership competencies if they are to meet the challenges of institutional transformation and system change. In particular, they need a system's perspective and competencies in developing strategic visions, risk taking, innovating and managing change. In our view this is where higher education and mentorship can make a fundamental and significant difference to the ways in which *experience* can be turned into *expertise* (see Rolfe 1998; Rolfe et al. 2001).

Ultimately, leadership development must be conceived as a lifelong process that encompasses multiple episodes of formal training that build upon prior professional experience. Individuals do learn from their experiences, but formal leadership development programmes facilitate focused self-assessment and mastery of new leadership competencies, well evidenced by Antrobus and her colleagues in Chapter 4. However, for the type of leadership development we have suggested in this chapter, perhaps a different approach is required.

Impact of globalization

Global development of a community for nurses and nursing leadership is imperative if the profession is to make the most of the experience, knowledge, and skills it has developed, as is also the case for AHPs. While, at present, there are numerous organizations flying an international flag, there is some criticism as to the extent that these groups are inclusive at an international level. For example, while exclusivity is often not intended, logistics are not always taken into account that an academic year does not run synchronously in the northern and southern hemispheres resulting in logistic, funding and attendance problems. Then there is the risk of developing a heavy organizational bureaucracy. As an organization expands globally, the challenge of managing such an extensive organization draws it away from the practice-based nurses and nursing leaders and makes it, per definition, elitist as it becomes accessible only to those in strategic positions.

Another challenge needing to be addressed is the great ethnocentric divide between Western and developing countries. Language barriers and hierarchical behaviour loom constantly on the horizon, reinforced as organizations are led and managed by an often shrinking core of people from the same country who are voted into office by their peers. This almost incestuous self-maintenance makes it difficult to introduce change and new ideas within the culture of the organization, and change is also often challenged by legislation.

With financial resources dwindling, it is becoming increasingly difficult to fund practitioners to attend international conferences and seminars, immediately excluding representation from developing countries – a phenomenon that reinforces the elitist perspective and excludes participation for the upcoming generation of nurses and nursing leaders. These are issues that present a direct challenge for twenty-first-century nursing leaders. One could envisage a community of leaders who not only could be prepared to develop communities of practice in various fields of nursing and health endeavour but also could be a community in itself, promoting knowledge and skill embedded in the subject of leadership. Such a community could span the globe and bring together the nursing community and organizations that could provide the visions, define the opportunities, and promote a broad and cosmopolitan outlook for nursing. This is a role that could be undertaken by such influential organizations as the International Council of Nurses, Colleges of Nursing and the nursing arm of the World Health Organization. Of course, each of these organizations also requires excellent leadership and vision.

Leading through communities of practice

Communities of practice are, to use a commonly referred-to definition, groups of people who share a concern, a set of problems, or a passion about a topic, and who deepen their knowledge and expertise in this area by interacting on an ongoing basis. They are a unique form of association, consisting of three core elements: a domain, which creates a common ground and a sense of identity; a community, which fosters interaction and the development of relationships; and a practice, the specific knowledge that the community develops, shares and maintains.

To these central components, it is possible to add a number of common characteristics. Thus, communities of practice should:

- Utilize productive enquiry
- Self-manage and self-govern
- Generate knowledge in support of their practice
- Assume accountability for supporting their members
- Collaborate via multiple channels
- Receive support from the organization, to varying degrees.

Achieving such a concept is a leadership challenge in itself. However, we suggest that only through the establishment of such a concept will nursing be able to activate its role in health care development and change.

We would argue that there is a need to hot-house or nurture leadership talent so that nurses can be better prepared for leadership roles, but in using this terminology be assured that we do not mean to educate leaders in a vacuum, rather through exposure to the real world, and through providing excellent and expert mentorship support. In the future the architecture of the nursing profession will be designed to incorporate the components of education, practice, administration policy and research. The unbundling of health care delivery into many more organizations and settings than has previously been the case is setting the stage for future health care. In Western societies the ongoing redesign, reorganization and restructuring in health care organizations is being driven by multiple events, including health care financing changes, quality improvement initiatives and shifting resources, accompanied by the constant development of health care technology and communication. New technologies and means of communication will eventually be viewed as a pathway to new definitions of care. And technological and communication changes will be seen as necessary to keep the growing bureaucracy in health care from restricting development of clinical services useful to patients.

Therefore one could postulate that the profession will have a common core of activities for continued development of its science, evaluation and improvement. Education, research and regulation will be specialized functions associated with universities, institutes, and virtual groups sharing the same specialties. Each nurse should be encouraged to develop a professional career profile in each of the five basic dimensions of nurses' professional role: education, practice, administration, policy and research awareness. Professional leadership in this scenario would be provided by nurses with doctoral degrees in one aspect of the full professional role. These nurses would be closely associated with professionals in other disciplines who share their areas of focus. An excellent example of nursing leadership in this form would be the late George Evers, who held professorial chairs in Belgium and Germany and was a clinical specialist in pain management running his own clinic. While teaching and undertaking research, he remained involved in professional organizations and nursing development at local, national and international levels.

Educators then may specialize in the delivery of basic and continuing education and would provide expertise in educational interventions for individuals and community health initiatives. They would be conversant with cognitive patterns and theories of learning. Using new technology to deliver education, designing curricula that can be used in local areas, they would coach and guide others in the use of learning materials and in educational processes. Institutions of education that centre on health care are complex adaptive systems and require educationalists to be familiar with and to apply the principles of complexity science, and approach which challenges the students' mental models and expanding their capacity for new actions. The concept of complexity science, specifically focuses on the principle of facilitating the students to reflect on and design their preferred futures – in other words support the individual to take control of and choreograph their personal future (Carter Kooken 2005). We would argue that leadership-based courses should be mindful of the concept of preferred futures in determining its content and approach. Designing preferred futures, according to complexity science, is a way of responding to current problems in an environment in which the future is not predictable. Certainly, as we have outlined thus far in this chapter, health care can be considered to be a large-scale unpredictable and complex institution in an unpredictable global environment. What we suggest is that energies in the present context are devoted to visioning what might be. In her interesting paper on nursing's preferred future, Carter Kooken (2005) identified the need to develop a 'future committee'. This group functioned as a formal knowledge-sharing network, managing and sharing knowledge 'related to the latest and predicted trends in society, health care and technology'. Moreover, Carter Kooken's team focused on a strategic objective that directly emphasized the role of nursing students in the development of health care leadership and suggest that:

> Nurse educators will consistently incorporate futuristic assignments and complexity science into coursework. Nursing students will learn to design preferred futures in order to become leaders in this profession.
>
> (Carter Kooken 2005)

This approach substantiates the idea of introducing leadership skills and experience throughout the undergraduate curriculum and as core module content in all further educational programmes.

Administrators and executives, in our view, should focus on resources and organization. Participating in the organizational design and operation of patient care delivery, ensuring that structures for patient care are relevant to patient requirements, the focus will be on design, decision making for effective use of resources, competency and outcomes. They will also engage in continual study of care delivery and outcomes, technology assessment, and development of ways to detect when changes should be planned and introduced, managing change and work with broad-based teams in all sectors of health care.

Policy experts will continue to be a major force in analysing public need for quality patient care and in ensuring that policy fosters health for all citizens. Nursing's policy experts will contribute to international, national and state policy initiatives in unique ways evidenced in patient care. To fulfil a strong patient advocacy role, nursing will establish a learning loop from the care experience to the policy table, as is well described through case studies in Chapter 5.

Researchers (and researcher practitioners) will of course continue to develop the science. They may be aligned with specific types of practices, and their research priorities will be to advance nurses' capability to provide quality patient care, but an important part of their role will be to make research findings accessible to practising nurses, facilitating application of research to practice. This approach to integrating research and practice is, in itself, a specialization demanding practical knowledge of applied research, excellent communication skills, expertise in the field of facilitation and the flexibility to remain focused on the needs of practising nurses, while incorporating challenges and introducing new ideas. In remaining practice-focused and communicating in a language at a level that is recognizable, such a person is a role model for practising nurses.

However, a word of caution, this structure and development could become disparate and unreconciled if leadership isn't exercised, and indeed it could be said that this is one of the profession's faults today, and has led to a disparate and weak body, not necessarily fulfilling it true potential in health care services. Each of these developments requires leadership in itself but how will we develop the overall leadership for nursing in the changing agenda of health care in the twenty-first century. Where do we find the new Nightingale? We contend that one approach is the establishment of communities of practice which we believe holds the means of achieving global leadership awareness and a way forward.

Leading for transformation: the importance of reflective processes for a community

Freshwater (2004) notes that, traditionally, leadership approaches tend towards the three-stage process of individual transformation (through self-directed learning), critical reflective and transformative learning. Leaders, have in the main, been taught to manage people. It is argued however, that twenty-first-century leadership demands that leaders motivate and manage movements to achieve long-lasting and sustainable change (Freshwater 2004; Sherwood and Freshwater 2005). Leading a movement that stimulates effective change requires a practitioner who is reflective and one who is willing to engage in a constant critical dialogue with their own and others' practices, emphasizing innovation and transformation. Transformational leadership based on reflective processes has the potential to capture the 'elusive, tacit quality of managing movement and dynamism' and requires constantly evolving individuals to facilitate it (Freshwater 2004: 22). Stanley's work (Chapter 7) attempts to refine the operational aspects of transformational leadership by articulating, what he calls, congruent leadership features. This presents an interesting discussion as it provides a potentially usable element of the specific; however, a word of caution that these features of transformational and congruent leadership are seen as complementary and are not placed in polarized positions – something nurses seem to excel at. It is true to say that challenging institutional attitudes demands a great deal of energy and commitment, as well as substantial support from peers and colleagues. Confronting organizational culture is both exciting and inspiring, but can also lead to disillusionment and despondency; hence we turn to our earlier comment on the significance of effective and expert mentorship. A supportive and reflective mentor will mirror back to the emerging leader their own vision for the organization that is intellectually rich, stimulating and rings true.

Conclusion

In summary, as Sherwood and Freshwater (2005) contend:

leadership that guides an organization through turbulent times must be able to break out of the box to see a new version of the present reality, thus viewing the workplace and its workers with a new lens.

(Sherwood and Freshwater 2005: 58)

As a silent majority nurses often assume that 'someone else will do it'. However, as we all know, each nurse has a responsibility to be a leader in shaping the environment. Adaptation of educational programmes and nurse education, we believe, should be exploring how any change process begins with the individual and expands in the circle of influence. This begins the process of developing transformational leaders – leaders who create lasting change (Bolman and Deal 2001). Transformational leaders create the possibility of building a culture that promotes the autonomy, communication and recognition that fosters a satisfied workforce. The workplace is transformed only as the leader transforms his or her own self, a nurturing spirit in the organization by inspiring individual workers to begin their own journey. Thus, educators are challenged to develop curricula models based on the emerging leader paradigm and move from the traditional transactional model towards one of transformation.

Key points

- Education is a key component of developing emerging leaders.
- Health care leaders require the skills of managing movement and dynamism as befitting a constantly evolving system.
- Leaders who aim to transform their practice inspire others to do the same.
- Transformative leaders lead through *expertise* as well as *experience*.
- If education is to develop transformational leaders fundamental changes are required in the thinking, delivery and philosophy of health care curricula.

Reflective exercises

1   Using your own experience and drawing upon the literature, reflect upon the role of education in inspiring and developing health care leaders. You may for example focus on the specific content of leadership programmes and the processes by which experienced and expert practitioners best learn. Other points for consideration include the influence of learning from experience, questions such as whether leadership skills can be taught or learnt and whether an individual needs to have the experience of having been in a leadership position to facilitate leadership skills in another person.

2   What sort of educational philosophy might best underpin a curriculum model designed specifically to develop dynamic and innovative health care leaders?

3   Spend some time reflecting on your understanding of the concept of transformational leadership and the notion of managing movement as opposed to people. How does this resonate with your own experience and with the wider picture of health care policy and practice?

4   Thinking around the concept of global communities of practice, how might the common characteristics defined earlier in this chapter translate into your own workplace? Are there ways in which the underpinning principles could be creatively adapted to enable you and your colleagues to engage in a productive enquiry around leadership skills and talents?

References

Alimo-Metcalfe, B. (1993) All snakes and no ladders. *Nursing Times* 89(38): 29–31.

Alimo-Metcalfe, B. (1995) An investigation of female and male constructs of leadership and empowerment. *Women in Management Review* 10(2): 3–8.

Bar-On, R. and Parker, J.D.A. (2000) (eds) *The Handbook of Emotional Intelligence*. San Francisco, CA: Jossey-Bass.

Bolman, L. and Deal, T. (2001) *Leading with Soul*. San Francisco, CA: Jossey-Bass.

Burnes, B. and Pope, R. (2007) Negative behaviours in the workplace: a study of two Primary Care Trusts in the NHS. *International Journal of Public Sector Management* 20(4): 285–303.

Carter Kooken, W.S. (2005) In pursuit of nursing's preferred future: through a new lens. *Reflections on Nursing Leadership* (downloaded on 28 March 2008 from http://nursingsociety.org/RNL/4Q_2005/features/feature4.html).

Cummings, G., Hayduk, L. and Estabrooks, C. (2005) Mitigating the impact of hospital restructuring on nurses: the responsibility of emotionally intelligent leadership. *Nursing Research* 54(1): 2–12.

Eagly, A.H. and Johannesen-Schmidt, M.C. (2001) The leadership styles of women and men. *Journal of Social Issues* 57(4): 781–797.

Esterhuizen, P. and Kooyman, A. (2001) Empowering moral decision making in nurses. *Nurse Education Today* 21: 640–647.

Farrell, G.A. (2001) From tall poppies to squashed seeds: why don't nurses pull together more? *Journal of Advanced Nursing* 35(1): 26–33.

Freshwater, D. (2000) Crosscurrents: against cultural narration in nursing. *Journal of Advanced Nursing* 32(2): 481–484.

Freshwater, D. (2004) A tool for clinical leadership. *Reflections on Nursing Leadership*. 30(2): 20–26.

Freshwater, D. and Robertson, C. (2002) *Emotions and Needs*. Buckingham: Open University Press.

Freshwater, D. and Stickley, T. (2004) The heart of the art: emotional intelligence in nursing. *Nursing Inquiry* 11(2): 91–98.

Goleman, D. (1995) *Emotional Intelligence*. New York: Bantam.

Herbert, R. and Edgar, L. (2004) Emotional intelligence: a primal dimension of nursing leadership? *Nursing Leadership* 7(4): 56–63.

House of Commons (2000) *Official Report (Hansard)* 22 March: cols 981–984: www.publications.parliament.uk/pa/cm199900/cmhansrd/cm000322/debtext/ 00322-04.htm#00322-04_spm.

James, A. (1998) Mary, Mary quite contrary, how do women leaders grow? *Women in Management Review* 13(2): 67–71.

Jasper, M.A. (1995) The potential of the professional portfolio for nursing ... maintenance and verification of continuing nursing practice following initial nursing training in the UK. *Journal of Clinical Nursing* 4(40): 249–255.

Kark, R. (2004) The transformational leader: who is (s)he? A feminist perspective. *Journal of Organizational Change Management* 17(2): 160–176.

Kim, M.J., Woith, W., Otten, K. and McElmurry, B.J. (2006) Global nurse leaders: lessons from the sages. *Advances in Nursing Science* 29(1): 27–42.

Kjervik, D.K. (1979) Women, nursing, leadership (editorial comment). *Image* 11(2): 34–36.

LCVV (Landelijk Centrum Verpleging en Verzorging) (2001) *Herregistratie van Basisverpleegkundigen: Een Literatuurstudie.* Utrecht: LCVV.

Madison, J. (1994) The value of mentoring in nursing leadership: a descriptive study. *Nursing Forum* 29(4): 16–23.

Mavin, S. (2006) Venus envy: problematizing solidarity behaviour and queen bees. *Women in Management Review* 21(4): 264–276.

Menzies-Lyth, I.E.P. (1970) *The Functioning of Social Systems as a Defence Against Anxiety.* London: Tavistock.

Menzies-Lyth, I.E.P. (1988) *Containing Anxiety in Institutions: Selected Essays.* London: Free Association Books.

Orbach, S. (1994) *What's Really Going on Here?* London: Virago.

Orbach, S. (1999) *Towards Emotional Literacy.* London: Virago.

Palmer, J. (2006) Testaments to mentoring. *Reflections on Nursing Leadership.* Honor Society of Nursing Sigma Theta Tau International. Third quarter 2006. Retrieved June 2008: http://nursingsociety.org/RNL/3Q_2006/features/feature4.html

Park, D. (1996). Gender role, decision style and leadership style. *Women in Management Review* 11(8): 13–17.

Ridgeway, C.L. (2001) Gender, status, and leadership. *Journal of Social Issues* 57(4): 637–655.

Rolfe, G. (1998) *Expanding Nursing Knowledge.* Oxford; Butterworth Heinemann.

Rolfe, G., Freshwater, D. and Jasper, M. (2001) *Critical Reflection for Health Care Professionals: A Users Guide.* Basingstoke: Palgrave.

Salvage, J. (2000) Doctors and nurses: doing it differently. The time is right for a major reconstruction. *British Medical Journal* 320: 1019–1020.

Sherwood, G. and Freshwater, D. (2005) Doctoral education for transformational leadership in a global context. In S. Ketefian and H. McKenna (eds) *Doctoral Education in Nursing: International Perspectives.* London: Routledge.

Skills for Health (2007) *Annual Review* Bristol: Department of Education and Skills.

Stickley, T. and Freshwater, D. (2002) The art of loving and the therapeutic relationship. *Nursing Inquiry* 9(4): 250–256.

Trinidad, C. and Normore, A.H. (2005) Leadership and gender: a dangerous liaison? *Leadership & Organization Development Journal* 26(7–8): 574–590.

Trossman, S. (1999) The professional portfolio: documenting who you are, what you do. *American Nurse* 31(2): 1–3.

Walsh, E. (2007) An examination of the emotional labour of nurses working in prison. Unpublished PhD thesis. Bournemouth University.

Yoder, J.D. (2001) Making leadership work more effectively for women. *Journal of Social Issues* 57(4): 815–828.

Further reading

Bolman, L.G. and Deal, T.E. (1997) *Reframing Organizations: Artistry, Choice, and Leadership*, 2nd edn. San Francisco, CA: Jossey-Bass.

Graham, I. (2003) Leading the development of nursing within a Nursing Development Unit: the perspectives of leadership by the team leader and a professor of nursing. *International Journal of Nursing Practice* 9(4): 213–222.

Kowalski, K. and Yoder-Wise, P. (2003) Five C's of leadership. *Nurse Leader* 1(5): 26–31.

Parker, M. and Gadbois, S. (2000) Building community in the healthcare workplace. *Journal of Nursing Administration* 30(9): 426–431.

Porter-O'Grady, T. and Malloch, K. (2003) *Quantum Leadership: A Textbook of New Leadership*. Boston, MA: Jones and Bartlett.

Salvage, J. (1987) *The Politics of Nursing*. London: Heinemann Nursing.

Sherwood, G.D. (2003) Leadership for a healthy work environment: caring for the human spirit. *Nurse Leader* 1(5): 36–40.

Trofino, J. (1995) Transformational leadership in health care. *Nursing Management* 20: 42–47.

Vitello-Cicciu, J.M. (2002) Exploring emotional intelligence: implications for nursing leaders. *Journal of Nursing Administration* 32(4): 203–210.

7 # Clinical leadership and the theory of congruent leadership

David Stanley

Overview

What are the qualities and characteristics of clinical leaders? Who are the clinical leaders? And why are some clinicians seen as clinical leaders and others, who might be expected to be seen as such, are not? This chapter explores these questions by outlining a research study designed to unpick the essentials of clinical leadership. From the results insights into clinical leadership are laid out and a new leadership theory – congruent leadership – is offered. This theory is explained in terms of its relevance to clinical leadership, and its potential to support and develop frontline leadership for nurses and other professional groups.

Introduction

In the United Kingdom clinical leadership has been the subject of considerable interest, and since 1997 the promotion of clinical leadership has intensified as the nursing profession and the National Health Service (NHS) recognized its value and promoted a greater role for nurses in the changing health service (Rafferty 1993; DoH 1998, 1999, 2000, 2004; Wedderburn-Tate 1999). Stronger nurse leadership has been described as 'crucial to the government's plans to modernise the NHS and to improve the public's health' (DoH 1999: 4). Mullally (2001: 24) suggested that 'strong nursing leadership is crucial if there is to be an effective nursing contribution' to the

UK government's change agenda. What was proposed was a new breed of clinical leader 'who can establish direction and purpose, inspire, motivate and empower teams around common goals and produce real improvements in clinical practice, quality and services' (DoH 1999: 52). As such the demand for leadership and specifically, a need to understand what constitutes clinical leadership has never been stronger (Chevannes 2000; Lett 2002).

However, if health care professionals are to have a significant impact on the development of clinical care and to the change agenda, discovering who the clinical leaders are and understanding the nature of clinical leadership is vital. This chapter addresses the following:

- What the qualities and characteristics of clinical leaders might be.
- Who the clinical leaders are.
- Why they are seen as clinical leaders.
- What the experience of clinical leadership might be.

This chapter also offers an introduction to a new leadership theory – congruent leadership. This leadership theory, developed from research related to clinical leadership, is offered as a new way to understand and develop clinical leadership for nurses and other health professionals.

Background

Discussions and research related to nursing leadership are not new, although it is only in recent years that clinical nurse leadership has featured more prominently in health-related literature. A wide sweep of topics includes empowerment, oppression, authority, power, management, the UK NHS political agenda, organizational structures, organizational cultures and boundaries between health professionals and their relationship to leadership roles within health care. A wealth of literature offered information that dealt with the role, nature and purpose of nursing leadership (see, for example, Scott 1987; Wright 1996; Antrobus and Kitson 1999; Footit 1999; McKeown and Thompson 1999; McKinnon 1999; Read 1999; Salvage 1999; Wedderburn-Tate 1999; Cunningham and Kitson 2000; Shepherd 2000; Faugier and Woolnough 2001; Nohre 2001; O'Neill 2001). Firth (2001) added further to the literature by describing the value of developing and nurturing nurse leaders. The work of McSherry and Browne (1997), Wedderburn-Tate (1999), Bower (2000), Cook (2001b), Chambers (2002), Crouch (2002) and McCormack and Garbett (2003) contributed further with a number of publications that addressed the characteristics or attributes of nurse leaders. However, very little literature of an empirical nature or of any depth addressed *clinical* leadership.

That said, a number of authors have attempted to describe the characteristics of nurse leaders, ward leaders and practice developers, who may be
considered broadly as 'clinical leaders' (Manley 1997, 2000a, 2000b; Christian and Norman 1998; Cosens et al. 2000; Cook 2001a, 2001b, 2001c; Guest
et al. 2001; Firth 2002; McCormack and Garbett 2003). These authors also
describe the primary role of a nurse leader or clinical nurse leader, suggesting
that it is to promote quality and to initiate and manage change. However, all
these studies (apart from Cook 2001a, 2001b, 2001c) described nurse leaders
at the higher end of the nursing hierarchy and as such propose that nursing
leadership and clinical nurse leadership require a broader or more eclectic
perspective for the leader to function effectively. Understanding the context
within which leadership takes place is important. Antrobus and Kitson
(1999) suggest that nursing leadership can better develop when nurses are
able to connect with the different parts of nursing, the political, the
academic, the managerial and the clinical domains; this is discussed in far
greater depth in Chapter 5. Christian and Norman (1998) and Firth (2002)
allude to this, but emphasize that broadening the role of the nurse leader can
also lead to conflict. This, it was suggested, results from the dual responsibilities of management and leadership which nursing leaders and clinical nurse
leaders often carry. It is also suggested that effective clinical leadership has a
direct impact on the standard of patient care and the values and principles
evident in the practice domain can therefore promote successful and lasting
change. Cosens et al. (2000) and Cook (2001a) discovered that when asking
questions about leaders or leadership, an appropriate place to begin was by
asking nurses and their peers and not to assume (based on hierarchical
structures) who the clinical leaders might be.

Significantly, while discussions of leadership are evident in a wide range of
nursing literature, much of it is focused on leadership from a management
perspective or on leadership of a general (not health specific) nature. Hurst
(1997), in the mid 1990s, also found that the theory and practice of nursing
leadership has been poorly developed and apart from anecdotal accounts,
little was written about nursing leadership in the UK until Rafferty (1993)
published a discussion paper that addressed nursing leadership issues. Here
she concluded, in relation to developing nursing's leadership potential, that:

> Getting it 'right' was less important than being prepared to take risks and
> make a start. It was felt important that different kinds of leadership were
> needed at different levels and times and therefore it was vital to have a
> pool of leaders upon which to draw. For this to happen, a number of
> different models of leadership needed to be fostered.
>
> (Rafferty 1993: 25)

Since Rafferty's appeal much has been achieved and different levels of
leadership have developed, although all appear to remain in what Antobus

and Kitson (1999: 751) call the 'academic, political and management domains'. Numerous studies and publications (Rafferty 1993; Antrobus and
Kitson 1999; McKeown and Thompson 1999; Faugier and Woolnough 2001;
Kitson 2001; Beech 2002; Firth 2002; Jasper 2002) have focused on nurse
leaders who hold senior posts either within organizations, nursing divisions,
wards and/or departments, and although clinical leadership is often mentioned, it is rarely the subject of research because of its low status (Antrobus
and Kitson 1999) when compared with other leadership domains. For this
reason the uniqueness of clinical leadership has remained largely unrecog-
nized and undervalued (Lett 2002). Indeed research specifically focusing on
clinical leadership is sparse and the term clinical leadership is often used
interchangeably and inappropriately, alongside or in conjunction with the
term nursing leadership (Lett 2002) or nursing management (Stanley 2006c).
This problem is compounded because much of the literature and research
related to nursing leadership has been developed to support nurses with
management responsibilities which has resulted in the principles of management being accepted as transferable when seeking insights or understanding
of other leadership areas. This widely held misconception, which is damaging to any real understanding of leadership, is discussed fully in Chapter 2.

A further reason for the slow development of different kinds of leadership
within nursing is that leaders have been sought who would support organizations that are trying to adapt and be successful in an environment of
constant organizational movement. This has resulted in leadership courses
and a vast amount of literature that invests solely in supporting change. This
is particularly the case for recent developments in the UK NHS, but this
applies across the globe as changes in health care delivery, the appearance of
new medical conditions (e.g. AIDS, SARS and Bird Flu) and advances in
medical technology have impacted on the delivery of health care and how
nurses have responded. In the UK, the United States and Canada advances in
technology have resulted in rapid changes in health care delivery models and
systems (McNeil 1995) and as such nursing leaders are required to adapt to
significant and constant changes. In all parts of the world, workforce issues,
such as an ageing nursing workforce and recruitment problems are impacting
on nurses' capacity to respond to care delivery needs leading to the
development of new roles and new ways of working. In Australia, New
Zealand, the UK, the United States and across the globe, nurses are being
asked to find ways to adapt to skilled nursing shortages (Australian Nursing
Federation 2008; Runy 2008; Wylie 2008).

These factors have led to a dependence on leadership theory that supports
change and understands leadership from the perspective of facilitating and
developing change. This required a theory where the followers could be
inspired and influenced towards a vision of some future state. With constant
change as a theme, nursing leadership programmes and the nursing profes-

sion's view of leadership have focused on an understanding of leadership based on the dominance of the transformational leadership theory and on the assumption that leaders must have 'vision' and influence or power to see their vision through. The NHS Confederation (1999: 4) supported this perspective when it indicated that, 'as the NHS seeks a new model for a new century, transformational leadership presents itself as an evidenced based technique'. In many respects this perspective is sound and for some levels and types of nursing leader or manager, this is the case. However, for other types of leadership, at different levels, this assumption may be counterproductive and inaccurate (Stanley 2008). The net effect is that Rafferty's (1993) suggestion that nursing needed to develop different leadership models for leaders at different levels has not been followed up, and consequently inappropriate or ineffective leadership models or theories dominate.

Defining leadership: leadership theories

Understanding the concept of leadership is pivotal to understanding the experiences of clinical nurse leaders and like Stogdill (1974: 7, cited in Crawford et al. 1997), who found that 'there are almost as many different definitions of leadership as there are people who have attempted to define the concept', studying leadership can be complicated by the plethora of definitions used to describe the term. Any literature search will show that there are numerous and often contradictory views on the meaning of leadership, however, for the purpose of exploring clinical leadership, an eclectic view of leadership is proposed where leadership is seen in terms of unifying people around values and then constructing the social world for others around those values and helping people get through change.

The fundamental concepts of leadership are discussed in Chapter 1; however, it is useful for the purposes of this chapter to consider those theories that pertain in particular to the caring professions. Work by Downton (1973), Burns (1978) and Bass (1985, 1990) described the transformational theory of leadership, which developed from an attempt to tease out the distinctions between management (associated with transactional leadership) and leadership (associated with transformational leadership). The latter is about challenging the status quo, creating a vision and sharing that vision, maintaining momentum and empowering others (Kakabadse and Kakabadse 1999). Day et al. (2000: 15) add to this perspective stating that 'transformational leaders not only manage structure, but they purposefully impact upon the culture in order to change it'. The transformational leader is not associated with status or power and is seen as being appropriate at all levels of an organization. The interdependence of followers and leaders within this theory has meant that transformational leadership has found favour in care related and teaching fields and, according to Welford (2002: 9), 'transformational leadership is arguably the most favourable leadership theory for clinical nursing in the general medical or surgical ward setting.' Thyer (2003: 73) also considers that it is 'ideologically suited to nurses', while Sofarelli and Brown (1998) indicate that it is a suitable leadership approach for empowering nurses. As mentioned earlier, the NHS Confederation (1999) indicates that transformational leadership is, in its view, best suited to modern leadership of the NHS. Subsequent work by George (2003: 12) takes the concept of caring further, describing the 'authentic leadership' theory, where leaders are guided by 'qualities of the heart, by passion, compassion' and lead 'with purpose, meaning and values'. Each theory has its merits, but are any of them useful or indeed relevant to an understanding of clinical leadership? Transformational theory may appear the most favourable theory for understanding clinical nursing, but has the reality of leading in the clinical environment or at the bedside been investigated to the point where any theory could be applied and used to develop a richer understanding of leadership that is not related to hierarchy, rank or position?

Research related to clinical leadership is sparse at best and it may be that one reason that clinical leaders have found it difficult to find their voice or exercise influence in the health arena is that they and others have not been able to articulate the type of leadership they offer (Stanley 2008). In order for clinical leaders to recognize their clinical leadership potential in both themselves and their colleagues it is essential that a leadership theory is established that supports the development of their skills and abilities as clinical nurse leaders. Theories help nurses and other health professionals contextualize their practice, giving it meaning and a foundation on which they can build their care and develop therapeutic relationships with their clients or patients. Likewise, clinical leadership may be best understood if our knowledge and insights of it are based on a theoretical foundation, or a paradigm, specifically related to clinical leadership. Currently contemporary leadership theories and frameworks, most of which have grown from the management domain, have neglected the reality and attributes associated with clinical leaders. Another, well-researched, perspective is needed to support and develop much needed clinical leadership.

New research

A research study (Stanley 2006a, 2006b) was carried out to identify the following:

- Who are the clinical leaders?
- Why are they seen as clinical leaders?
- What are the experiences of a clinical leader?

The study approach was fundamentally qualitative in nature, based on a grounded theory (Glaser and Strauss 1967; Chenitz and Swanson 1986; Glaser 1992; Strauss and Corbin 1998) and employed questionnaires, interviews and casual observations to generate data. The organization recruited to the study was a large acute UK NHS trust that was able to cater for nearly one thousand inpatients in a wide variety of clinical specialities, and offered extensive outpatient, diagnostic and support facilities. The research approach was divided into three phases:

1   A questionnaire sent to qualified nurses in all the principal patient care areas with the aim of identifying the qualities and characteristics associated with clinical leaders and exploring who the clinical leaders were in each of the clinical areas surveyed.
2   In-depth, semi-structured and focused interviews to explored issues related to perceptions of clinical leadership and to discover which staff where seen as clinical leaders.
3   Identifying and interviewing two of the clinical leaders nominated by the majority of the participants interviewed in phase two, from each of the four clinical areas.

Characteristics and qualities of clinical leaders

Participants in the study identified the 'most' and 'least' attributes in the questionnaire as indicated in Table 7.1.

Table 7.1 Characteristics and qualities 'most' and 'least' associated with clinical leadership

MOST	LEAST
Approachable (97.3%)	Controlling (78.1%)
Clinically competent (95.2%)	Artistic (65.9%)
Motivator (94.1%)	Conservative (62.2%)
Supportive (94.1%)	Routine (57.4%)
Inspires confidence (93.0%)	Calculator (47.3%)
Copes well with change (90.9%)	Reward/punishment (39.3%)
Flexibility (90.4%)	Administrator (33.5%)
Sets direction (89.3%)	Regulator (32.4%)
Directing and helping (88.8%)	Aligns people (27.1%)
Integrity (82.2%)	Maintenance (25.0%)

Participants added a number of other qualities or characteristics associated with clinical leadership, indicating that clinical leaders have current clinical practice skills, for example, 'do the same thing as the staff they lead' and 'mucks in and works on all levels'. Many of the additions related to interpersonal and communication skills or attitudes appropriate for a clinical leader, such as 'good listener', 'hard working', 'understanding', 'honest' and 'reliable'. Some referred to their clinical leader's relationship to their team or to other health care workers, for example, 'ability to unite a team/group' and 'looks out for the best interests of the team' and some related to the caring aspects of the clinical leaders role 'puts patient care first', 'compassion' and 'caring'.

In 2007 a follow-up study was undertaken opportunistically with a group of final semester nursing students in Australia. They were offered and completed the same questionnaire and generated results principally in keeping with the primary study. Australian nursing students indicated that the key characteristics of clinical leaders were:

- Approachability
- Clinical competence
- Copes well with change
- Flexibility supportive
- Motivator
- Inspirational, inspires confidence
- Critical thinking.

Critical thinking was identified as a characteristic included by the Australian nurses and was the only notable difference. In conversations with the Australian respondents it appeared that critical thinking was seen as a skill or attribute that supported clinical competence, and respondents were simply reinforcing the dominant characteristic of clinical competence. 'Controlling' was again rated as the characteristic least associated with the qualities of a clinical leader, aligning this data comfortably with the initial questionnaire results from the UK.

Clinical leaders it seemed were not managers. Or at least, not managers who were away from the clinical area, who were unapproachable, not seen as clinically competent or able to motivate and inspire their staff. To be recognized as a clinical leader meant thinking critically and acting in clinical practice in a way that clinical colleagues associated with the values and principals of clinical practice. Further exploration as to the participants' understanding of the attributes and qualities that make good or, indeed, poor leaders indicated that many of the participants considered it a leader's responsibility to empower people to perform better. One participant said, 'It's about getting the best out of people.' Most participants described leaders as guides and teachers, indicating that they should be open, approachable and get people to feel part of a team. Many suggested that a leader should provide support, motivate and be someone whom they could look up to or admire. Leaders held a central role in the clinical area and were described as having drive or as being assertive. Clinical leaders were also described as being the 'figurehead', and 'beacon' in the clinical area. Effective clinical leaders were also seen as taking responsibility, communicating well, having sound knowledge, being inspirational and were considered to be "really approachable ... really looked out for you".

Clinical leaders were seen to be effective and respected because they had 'some sort of belief in themselves', or were able to stand up for what they believe; they were nurses at all levels who promoted, defended or stood up for high standards of patient care. It soon became apparent that clinical leadership was less associated with titles, positions, grades and responsibilities, and more related to the beliefs and values a nurse held about fulfilling their duties and responsibilities. This perspective was summed up by one participant, who said:

> "I think you've got to have respect for that person [clinical leader] because of the way they nurse, you identify with them, identify with the way they nurse and agree with that."

Negative clinical leadership qualities and characteristics were associated with gossiping, moodiness, not listening and laziness. This was summed up by one participant, who said poor clinical leaders were:

> "Indecisive, fail to keep up with their knowledge, don't listen to anybody, are not open to questions, 'Why do you do this?' 'Well we just always do it that way.' It just doesn't help ... people that are 'hidebound' (sit down a lot) or people that have to always be right, or who are not open to questions or people that just don't do the work ... lazy people ... pen pushers ... people that sit in the office all the time."

They were also perceived as often having a dictatorial attitude, no sense of humour, were bullies, or were described as 'out of control and not aware of what was going on'. Others were unapproachable, uninterested, disorganized, 'laid back' or showed favouritism towards particular colleagues. Nurses who lacked communication skills, or worked to their own agendas, or 'didn't appear to be out there doing clinical nursing' were also criticized.

Clinical leadership attributes

The characteristics and qualities strongly associated with clinical leadership were identified as *clinical competence*, which related to remaining credible and competent. It meant being able to show, or to do, as well as know or teach others about clinical issues. One participant said, 'Clinically you need to be having some input otherwise you lose your credibility.'

Clinical knowledge or knowledge of nursing that related to a specific clinical area of practice was vital. This was extended into knowing not just about clinical issues, but knowing about teamwork, how individuals worked and of interpersonal relationships. One participant said, 'You've got to be knowledgeable, but you've also got to have knowledge that's applicable to the area that you work in.' Another added, 'You have to be a clinical expert in your field ... and you have to have gone through that process from novice to expert.'

Effective communication was seen as a central attribute of clinical leadership. Clinical leaders were respected if they listened and effective communication was seen as elemental if clinical leaders who were not managers or titled leaders were to influence their colleagues. They needed to be 'Extremely good at explaining things at the right level that you understand' and 'The ward manager has got the title and therefore they manage and are seen to be leaders because of the title, but there are other people that lead by virtue of their opinion.'

Decision making, not just in relation to patient care or clinical issues, but in regard to a whole host of issues was considered important to clinical leadership. Allied to this was the ability to delegate and problem-solve.

Effective clinical leadership was considered to be aligned with *empowerment* or *motivation*. It involved being enthusiastic, being able to make colleagues feel confident, supported and encouraged. It was also seen to be about empowering people to perform better, sowing a seed somewhere and letting others take the lead. One participant described it as a 'belief in what you're doing ... because I know people who are higher, at a higher level than me are not necessarily good leaders ... they're not ... they don't necessarily have any belief in what they're doing'.

Openness and *approachability* were seen as desirable characteristics and qualities of clinical leaders. Many participants looked for clinical leaders who 'valued them', were 'approachable, friendly and understanding', or who were 'open, caring', 'knowledgeable, fair, tranquil, calm, kept secrets' or whom 'you could talk to about anything'. Clinical leaders were identifiable because, unlike managers, they were viewed by participants as *role models*. They had their standards of care on show and other nurses indicated that it was the ability of a nurse to care effectively for their patients that made them stand out as a clinical leader. They were seen as 'Someone you would look up to' and 'people that have been inspirational or people you've thought, "Oh that's what I really want to be like".'

Linked to the concept of being a role model was the attribute of *visibility*. Clinical leaders were identifiable because a significant part of their role involved engaging directly in patient care and any post or role that limited contact with or relationships with patients or clients would limit their ability to act out, or live out their values or beliefs and limit others ability to recognize them as clinical leaders. It was apparent from the questionnaire and interview data that the values and principles a clinical leader displayed were a prominent aspect of their identification, and that the values and beliefs that a clinical leader displayed were a key factor in their being recognized as a clinical leader. Describing clinical leaders, one participant said, 'They've really got this passion and belief about what they do and why they are here.'

This work indicated that clinical leaders were recognized because they were 'discoverers', 'enablers', 'shapers' (with 'creativity' to generate new ways of working) and 'modifiers' who supported and helped others with the process of change. The characteristics described above are in keeping with many of Cook's findings because both describe clinical leaders as knowing and being able to do the work central to their clinical area and practice role. A significant difference between Cook's (2001b) study and the results outlined here are that Cook saw clinical leaders as 'creative', identifying the typology of 'shapers' to describe them, a difference also identified by Rolfe (2006), and found again in the replication study in Australia. However, *critical thinking*, which may be strongly linked to creativity, was ranked very highly, perhaps leaving the door ajar to a link between creativity and the attributes identifiable with clinical leaders.

Antrobus and Kitson (1999: 750) identified 'understanding self and having a clear understanding of values, purpose and personal meaning' as part of the skills repertoire they identified for effective nurse leaders. This is in keeping with Cook (2001b) who saw clinical nurse leaders as 'valuers', empathizing with others and gauging their own and others' feelings, a view supported by McCormack and Garbett (2003), who indicated that 'practice developers' valued and strove for an emotional engagement with their work. The evidence available suggests that clinical leaders are driven by their values and a 'passion' for high quality patient care, and in displaying these principles they stand apart.

They were followed, therefore, not for their vision and creativity (although they may have had these attributes), or because they were in positions of control, but because they were role models for their values and beliefs – it was these that were on show and evident in their actions.

Who are the clinical leaders?

The results of this study indicated that junior registered nurses and sisters were most likely to be viewed as clinical leaders by their colleagues, and although modern matrons and nurse managers were acknowledged to be in senior positions, their effectiveness and validity as clinical leaders can be challenged by the results. In one interview the interviewee pointed to a colleague to make her point: 'There, that one. Yes, the one by the bed. If my mum gets sick or is admitted here, that's who I want to have look after her.' Clinical leaders were identified because they were more focused on the 'clinical' than on the 'leadership' emphasis of their role. Nurses in management positions were not seen as clinical leaders, and were rarely nominated as such by those questioned. Instead, frontline, clinically engaged nurses were most often seen as the clinical leaders.

It is interesting to note that frontline, clinical staff are rarely the subject of leadership studies or are evident in nursing leadership literature. It may be that clinical nurses have been unrecognizable as clinical leaders because most function at the bedside doing 'nursing work'. Doing what Robinson (1992) and Davies (1995) called the 'invisible' and what Roberts (1983) and Wilkinson and Miers (1999) called the 'dirty' work of nursing. This invisibility is compounded because clinical leaders are often measured against a set of criteria, characteristics and qualities more in keeping with general leadership or management ideologies and attributes. Leadership courses too often feature programmes that while titled 'leadership' look more like management courses and are rarely offered or suitable for frontline clinical staff. Management and leadership are different (Stanley 2006c) and until clinical leaders are identified and recognized (and indeed recognize themselves), much of the leadership investment made by organizations will miss its mark and fail to support the development of quality health services.

The experience of being a clinical leader

Some of the clinical leaders identified were surprised to be nominated, a finding consistent with the Delphi study carried out by Butterworth and Bishop (1995) on best clinical practice. This poses the question, does this indicate a lack of recognition of the importance of enhanced clinical practice from the nursing hierarchy? Those that responded with surprise were all junior registered nurses or sisters and it appeared that they were surprised because the focus for their role was related to patient care and not management or administrative duties – shadows of the subordinate and invisible position of 'nursing work' cast across their comments (Wilkinson and Miers 1999). The clinical leaders described the majority of their role as being related to the delivery of hands-on patient care and well prepared for their role because of their clinical experience, giving them credibility in their clinical field. They all spoke passionately about their involvement in patient care and how they 'thrived on client contact'. They saw themselves and they felt others saw them as clinical leaders because of their 'visibility ... the fact that I am out there doing it every day'.

Another avenue for understanding clinical leadership related to the challenges that clinical leaders faced. The first and most dominant challenge related to conflict between their leadership and management functions. Many interviewees indicated that they found that their managerial responsibilities were very much in conflict with their leadership responsibilities, with one admitting that she was 'desperately, desperately trying to keep as hands on as possible' by taking management work home or delegating part of it to other staff. These comments appeared to be particular to participants who held senior nursing posts or who were able to express an insight into the duality of their management or leadership role. The perception that the 'negative side of nursing promotion is a greater tendency to come off the shop floor' and that this can 'diminish your impact as a clinical leader' led to considerable conflict; indeed some had made a conscious decision not to advance their career further as their clinical expertise would be submerged under management duties. The second challenge related to difficulties with keeping staff motivated so that the patients continued to receive the best care. Clinical leaders commonly found themselves with limited ability to influence the health service or even their own clinical area.

These challenges are not new and they highlight discussions within nursing that draw attention to the tension between some nurses' clinical leadership responsibilities and management function (Rafferty 1993; Christian and Norman 1998; Antrobus and Kitson 1999; Firth 2002; McCormack and Garbett 2003; Thyer 2003, Stanley 2006c). The challenge commonly felt was one that pulled clinical leaders between their desire to remain clinically focused and demands to maintain the management and resource capabilities of their clinical area. Pendleton and King (2002: 1354) called this the 'ethos gap'. The clinical leaders cited above confirmed that leadership and management were different things and that it is inappropriate to base an understanding of clinical leadership on theories, frameworks and models that have developed from – and are best suited to – business and management functions. To do so can offer only an inadequate and incomplete insight into how best to promote, understand or develop clinical, practice–based leadership. As a result, *congruent leadership* is proposed as a new framework that satisfies and accommodates all the qualities and characteristics recognized as attributable to clinical leaders and meets the needs of clinical nurse leaders to be seen and valued for the often invisible, but vital contribution they make.

Congruent leadership

Congruent leadership theory can be seen when the clinical leaders' activities, actions and deeds are matched by and driven by their values and beliefs about (in this case) care and nursing. They may have a vision, be creative and have an idea about where they want to go, but this is not why they are followed; *they are effective because their leadership is based on shared values, beliefs and principles*. In addition, congruent leaders were considered motivational, inspirational, organized, effective communicators and built effective relationships, in many ways mirroring the skills necessary to develop effective therapeutic clinical relationships. Many have no formal, recognized or hierarchical leadership position and as such congruent leadership may offer a better theoretical framework to explain how and why they function, and clarify why and how non-titled leaders at all levels can function and be effective: Table 7.2 compares the features of congruent and transformational leadership. One clinical leader summed this up, saying:

> Honesty, loyalty, passion, integrity those sort of things are probably more important ... years ago when I was less experienced I would have said knowledge would have been oh, right up there, but because of the way I have changed, I don't think that this is necessarily so any more ... these other qualities outweigh them.

Table 7.2 A comparison of the features of transformational and congruent leadership

TRANSFORMATIONAL LEADERSHIP FEATURES	CONGRUENT LEADERSHIP FEATURES
Establishing direction	Motivating and inspiring
Aligning people	Approachable/open
Motivating and inspiring	About where you stand (principles)
Produces change – often dramatic	Actions based on values and beliefs
About where you are going (vision)	Effective communicators
Effective communicators	Visible
Creative / initiative	Empowered

NB: Although there are some similarities the key differences relate to what motivates the leaders: vision or values and principles.

An example of congruent leadership in action can be seen in the case study.

Case study 7.1 Ward open?

A junior qualified nurse was faced with an anxious husband whose wife had undergone emergency surgery. The husband wanted to visit his wife and be at her side, following her surgery, but he had to work when the ward had visiting times. The ward enforced strict visiting times for all relatives and other visitors and although the ward was 'open' for a number of hours, this man was unable to attend at these times. The nurse, knowing she was acting against the specific instructions of the ward manager and senior sister, allowed the man onto the ward at a 'closed' time to visit his wife. The nurse allowed this course of action because she believed that had this been her husband or had she been the wife, this was the action she would have wanted the nurse to follow. The nurse knew that she could have incurred the disapproval of the ward managers, and indeed did so; the fallout from her action was that she was reprimanded. However, this event initiated debate at the regular ward meeting that ultimately resulted in many of this nurse's colleagues agreeing that they would have liked to have done the same and this, in time, led to a revision in the ward's visiting processes and procedures. The nurse had no long-term strategy in mind; she simply followed her beliefs about respecting the needs of patients and their relatives. This event initiated what developed into a slow revolution that resulted in significant change and an improvement in the access that relatives enjoyed to their ill, worried and isolated friends and family.

Followers are attracted to congruent leaders because of the banner or standard they carry. They may not even intentionally show it or they may not be conscious that others see it, but it is this that followers recognize and rally to. Their metaphorical banner or standard is usually a statement of what the clinical leader believes is important to them. It might say 'I care for patients like they were my family.' 'I teach these children as if they were my own.' 'I'll be here at the bedside with you.' 'I know what it's like' or 'I'm on your side.' This is in accord with the work of Manley (2000a, 2000b), who was successful as a clinical leader because others saw her values on show. Her values supported and matched her actions and this congruence formed the basis for her success as a clinical leader. Manley (2000b) recognized that her leadership brought about 'cultural change' because her values were used to 'highlight the contradiction between espoused culture and culture in practice' (Manley 2000b: 34). She identified her leadership style as transformational because it was her aim to affect and change the culture of the unit.

However, when reading the examples given by respondents in Manley's research it is clear that they were influenced more by her actions than by her vision. One said, 'the enthusiasm of the consultant nurse incited enthusiasm in myself' (quoted in Manley 2000b: 37).

Taking an overall view of professional leadership, Roberts (1983) indicated that it may be necessary to view current nursing leadership with scepticism because nursing leaders, in order to break free from oppression, adopt the leadership attributes of the oppressors. In so doing they become unwitting or even complicit co-oppressors, who through their approach to leadership and educational structures support the status quo, maintaining or relegating nurses and nursing to a second-class or subservient status. This approach to leadership leads to divisiveness and competition among nurses and to avoid this, Roberts (1983: 29) suggested that elite leadership should be shunned and nursing should aim to develop leadership from the grassroots perspective. In many respects this is what Manley was able to achieve, as her colleagues became more empowered and emancipated as 'practitioners become aware of their values, beliefs and assumptions and helping them to act on them' (Manley 2000b: 38). In effect Manley's research and the example offered are centred on grassroots leadership that is in keeping with the principles of congruent leadership.

If clinical health care professionals are to develop effective clinical leaders, they need to do so without losing the core values and principles that guide patient care. Congruent leadership establishes a foundation from which all good or effective clinical leaders can start, because it grounds the leader's principles within the core values of the 'caring professions', ensuring that the dominant cultural narrative is one of patient-centred care, with care-centred attributes placed ahead of those associated with the dominant (potentially) oppressor groups of managers and physicians. Transformational leaders, in an effort to achieve their vision or goals, could at times, move from positions of influence and power to positions of control. Unwittingly, in doing so, they run the risk of losing their connection to their core values and guiding principles, or at best become embroiled in a state of conflict as their managerial (controlling) demands conflict with their professional and often personal desire to remain focused on patient care.

Congruent leadership is not power neutral; the power of congruent leadership comes from unifying groups and individuals around common values and beliefs. Nurses generally spend the most time with patients of all health professionals, and nurses who seek to lead in a clinical environment will find greater success if their values and beliefs are consistent with the dominant values and beliefs of their colleagues or if they are able to bring their colleagues to a point where their values and beliefs about care coincide. Conflict can result if the principles and values of one group or individual are at odds with others and power and influence in terms of leading falls often to the dominant group or leader. While transformational leaders derive their power and influence from being able to articulate a vision that is accepted and acted upon by the majority of the followers, congruent leaders' power and influence is derived from being able to articulate and display their values, beliefs and principles.

In support of this view of congruent leadership a passage from Hankey's 'The Beloved Captain' is offered. In it he describes an infantry officer in the trenches of the First World War. Junior officers at the Front took considerable risks along with the men they led, unlike the 'Chateau Generals' miles behind the lines and safe from the frontline action! Like clinical leaders, these junior officers were visible, present and linked to the men in the trenches by the values and beliefs they held. Hankey describes one such officer as:

> Tall, erect, smiling … for a few days he just watched. Then he started work. He picked out some of the most awkward ones and … marched them away by themselves … His confidence was infectious … His simplicity could not fail to be understood … very soon the awkward squad found themselves awkward no longer … The fact was that he had won his way into our affections. We loved him … If anyone had a sore foot he would kneel down and look at it. If a blister had to be lanced, he would very likely lance it himself … There was something almost religious about this care for our feet. It seemed to have a touch of the Christ about it.
>
> (Hankey 1917, cited in Keegan 1996: 275–276)

It is the officer's ability to get down on his knees, put his beliefs into action, be approachable, visible and caring, and communicate skilfully with the men that allows him to win over his followers with 'affection'. These are the actions of a frontline, hands-on congruent leader. Successful clinical leadership is therefore proposed to rest on a model that is based on leaders who respond to challenges and critical problems with actions and activities in accordance with (congruent with) their values and beliefs. The strengths of congruent leadership are that it supports the promotion of grassroots (Roberts 1983) leaders. It offers a foundation for other theories of leadership to be built upon. No longer invisible, the value of direct patient care work can be recognized and clinical leaders can have a positive impact, and lead by standing by the principles central to their profession.

While it is posited that congruent leadership may offer nurses and frontline clinical professionals an opportunity to develop greater influence in the leadership stakes, until health professionals *themselves* can recognize and initiate this and see themselves as congruent leaders, others will continue to see clinical work as 'dirty' and 'invisible' (Roberts 1983; Robinson 1992; Davies 1995; Wilkinson and Miers 1999) and clinical staff will remain of low status (Antrobus and Kitson 1999), invisible and dirty by association. As with Hankey's officer, congruent leadership is not static, but dynamic. It is not just about being, but about acting, displaying, demonstrating, living the leader's values and beliefs. The result of congruent leadership is a change or identification with the culture of a group or organization rather than simply addressing group structure as it represents a new perspective on clinical leadership and is helpful for advancing an understanding of clinical leadership.

Conclusion

Congruent leaders build their approach to clinical leadership on a foundation of care that is fundamental to their view of how patients should be cared for. Clinical leadership is commonly demonstrated in the ward or unit, by a person who is directly involved in providing care, by staff who are visible to their colleagues and considered to be knowledgeable and competent. Leaders who control and manage from within offices or who fail to display their values and beliefs in congruence with their actions are rarely seen as clinical leaders.

This chapter adds to an understanding of clinical leadership, and indicators have been found that point toward the significant contribution clinical leaders can make if they are recognized as such and encouraged to see that leadership does indeed exist at many levels. Clinical leaders commonly display *congruent leadership* and their passion for participation in hands-on patient care and in striving to contribute to high quality nursing adds to the pool from which nursing leaders can be drawn. However, they need to be recognized as such, by themselves and the profession in general, because the nurse leader who stands by what they believe is as valuable and as effective, as the leader with the grand plan.

Key points

- Clinical leaders are present in large numbers and at all levels of clinical practice.
- Current theories of leadership may be insufficient to support an understanding of clinical leadership.
- Clinical leaders can be recognized because they are clinically competent, cinically knowledgeable, effective communicators, decision makers, empowered motivators, open and approachable, role models and visible.
- Clinical leaders are mostly likely not to be managers and are commonly the most senior level of clinically engaged staff level (e.g. F Grade Nurse or Clinical Nurse).
- Congruent leadership is proposed as a suitable and effective theory to support and explain clinical leadership.

Reflective exercises

1   Look about your clinical environment. Who would you identify as a clinical leader? Make a list of their names, roles and position description. Why did you select this person or people?
2   What characteristics or attributes do you look for in a clinical leader?
3   Find out a little about the work of both Mary Seacole and Florence Nightingale in the Crimea. Jot down a few points related to their clinical roles in this war. Based on what has been described in this chapter, who might you identify as a congruent leader? It might be that they both fit the bill, but what was it about them that set them apart?
4   Think about your own practice. Would you describe yourself as a transformational or congruent leader? Which theory best supports your view of clinical leadership?

References

Australian Nursing Federation (2008) Media Release: Australian Nursing Federation. MediaNet Press Release Wire, Sydney, 8 June.

Antrobus, S. Kitson, A. (1999) Nursing leadership: influencing and shaping health policy and nursing practice. *Journal of Advanced Nursing* 29(3): 746–753.

Bass, B.M. (1985) *Leadership and Performance Beyond Expectations*. New York: Free Press.

Bass, B.M. (1990) From transactional to transformational leadership: learning to share the vision. *Organisational Dynamics* 18: 19–31.

Beech, M. (2002) Leaders or managers: the drive for effective leadership. *Nursing Standard* 16(30): 35–36.

Bower, F.L. (2000) *Nurses Taking the Lead*. Philadelphia, PA: Saunders.

Burns, J.M. (1978) *Leadership*. New York: Harper and Row.

Butterworth, T. Bishop, V. (1995) Identifying the characteristics of optimum practice: findings from a survey of practice experts in nursing, midwifery and health visiting. *Journal of Advanced Nursing* 22: 24–32.

Chambers, N. (2002) Nursing leadership: the time has come to just do it. *Journal of Nursing Management* 10: 127–128.

Chenitz, C.W. Swanson, J.M. (1986) *From Practice to Grounded Theory: Qualitative Research in Nursing*. Wokingham: Addison-Wesley.

Chevannes, M. (2000) On the right track. *Nursing Management* 7(6): 18–20.

Christian, S.L. and Norman, I.J. (1998) Clinical leadership in Nursing Development Units. *Journal of Advanced Nursing* 27: 108–116.

Cook, M. (2001a) Clinical leadership that works. *Nursing Management* 7(10): 24–28.

Cook, M. (2001b) The attributes of effective clinical nurse leaders. *Nursing Standard* 15(35): 33–36.

Cook, M. (2001c) The renaissance of clinical leadership: International Council of Nursing. *International Nursing Review* 48: 38–46.

Cosens, M., Ibbotson, T. Grimshaw, J. (2000) Identifying opinion leaders in ward nurses: a pilot study. *Journal of Research in Nursing* 5(2): 148–155.

Crawford, M., Kydd, L. and Riches, C. (eds) (1997) *Leadership and Teams in Educational Management*. Buckingham: Open University Press.

Crouch, D. (2002) Leading lights. *Nursing Times* 98(15): 24–26.

Cunningham, G. Kitson, A. (2000) An evaluation of the RCN Clinical Leadership Development Programme: Part 2. *Nursing Standard* 15(13–15): 34–40.

Davies, C. (1995) *Gender and the Professional Predicament in Nursing*. Buckingham: Open University Press.

Day, C., Harris, A., Hadfield, M., Tolley, H. Beresford, J. (2000) *Leading Schools in Times of Change*. Buckingham: Open University Press.

Department of Health (1998) *A First Class Service: Quality in the New NHS*. London: Stationary Office.

Department of Health (1999) *Making a Difference*. London: Stationary Office.

Department of Health (2000) *The NHS Plan*. London: Stationary Office.

Department of Health (2004) *National Standards, Local Action: Health and Social Care Standards and Planning Framework 2005–2007/8*. London: Stationary Office.

Downton, J.V. (1973) *Rebel Leadership: Commitment and Charisma in a Revolutionary Process*. New York: Free Press.

Faugier, J. Woolnough, H. (2001) At face value – shutting nurse managers out of top jobs. *Health Service Journal* 6: 24–29.

Firth, K. (2001) Developing the nurse leaders of the future. *Professional Nurse – Supplement* 16(8): S5–S6.

Firth, K. (2002) Ward leadership: balancing the clinical and managerial roles. *Professional Nurse* 17(8): 486–489.

Footit, B. (1999) Leading nurses into the future. *Nursing Management* 6(2): 23–26.

George, B. (2003) *Authentic Leadership: Rediscovering the Secrets of Creating Lasting Value*. San Francisco, CA: Jossey-Bass.

Glaser, B.G. (1992) *Basics of Grounded Theory Analysis*. Mill Valley, CA: Sociology Press.

Glaser, B.G. Strauss, A.L. (1967) *The Discovery of Grounded Theory*. New York: Aldine.

Guest, D., Peccei, R., Rosenthal, P., Montgomery, J., Redfern, S., Young, C., Wilsons-Barnet, J., Dewe, P., Evans, A. and Oakley, P. (2001). *A Preliminary Evaluation of the Establishment of Nurse Midwife and Health Visitor Consultants*. London: Department of Health and King's College London.

Hankey, D. (1917) The beloved captain. In D. Hankey, *A Student in Arms: Selected Essays*. New York: E.P. Duttton.

Hurst, K. (1997) *A Review of the Nursing Leadership Literature: Nuffield Institute*. Leeds: University of Leeds.

Jasper, M. (ed.) (2002) Nursing roles and nursing leadership in the new NHS – changing hats same heads. *Journal of Nursing Management* 10: 63–64.

Kakabadse, A. Kakabadse, N. (1999) *Essence of Leadership*. London: International Thomson Business Press.

Keegan, J. (1996) *The Face of Battle*. London: Pimlico.

Kitson, A. (2001) Nursing leadership: bringing caring back to the future. *Quality in Health Care*. 10(Supplement 11): ii79–ii84.

Lett, M. (2002) The concept of clinical leadership. *Contemporary Nurse* 12(1): 16–20.

McCormack, B. Garbett, R. (2003) The characteristics and skills of practice developers. *Journal of Clinical Nursing* 12(3): 317–325.

McKeown, C. Thompson, J. (1999) Learning the art of management. *Nursing Management* 6(5): 8–11.

McKinnon, B. (1999) Leadership: a means of empowering the nursing profession. *Contemporary Nurse* 8(1): 252–254.

McNeil, B. (1995) Implementing advances in medical technology: the American view. *Journal of the Royal Society of Medicine* 88(Supplement 26): 26–27.

McSherry, R. Browne, J. (1997) Tools of the trade. *Nursing Times*, Leadership Supplement 93(25).

Manley, K. (1997) A conceptual framework for advanced practice: an action research project operationalising an advanced practitioner/consultant nurse role. *Journal of Clinical Nursing* 6: 190–197.

Manley, K. (2000a) Organisational culture and consultant nurse outcomes: Part 1, Organisational culture. *Nursing Standard* 14(36): 34–38.

Manley, K. (2000b) Organisational culture and consultant nurse outcomes: Part 2, Nurse outcomes. *Nursing Standard* 14(37): 34–39.

Mullally, S. (2001) Leadership and politics. *Nursing Management* 8(4): 21–27.

NHS Confederation (1999) *Consultation: The Modern Values of Leadership and Management in the NHS.* London: NHS Confederation and Nuffield Trust.

Nohre, A. (2001) Soul + Spirit + Resources + Leadership = Results. *Journal of Nursing Administration* 3(6): 287–289.

O'Neill, S. (2001) Clinical governance in action. *Professional Nurse* 16(10): 1396–1397.

Pendleton, D. King, J. (2002) Values and leadership: education and debate. *British Medical Journal* 325: 1352–1355.

Rafferty, A.M. (1993) *Leading Questions: a Discussion Paper on the Issues of Nurse Leadership.* London: King's Fund Centre.

Read, C. (1999) Clinical leadership experience for the beginning nursing student. *Nurse Educator* 24(4): 7–8.

Roberts, S.J. (1983) Oppressed group behaviour: implications for nursing. *Advances in Nursing Science* 5: 21–30.

Robinson, J. (1992) Introduction: beginning the study of nursing policy. In J. Robinson, A. Gray and R. Elkan (eds) *Policy Issues in Nursing.* Buckingham: Open University Press.

Rolfe, G. (2006) Review: in command of care. Toward the theory of congruent leadership. *Journal of Research in Nursing* 2(20): 145–146.

Runy, L.A. (2008) The aging workforce. *Hospital and Health Networks* 82(1) 49–53.

Salvage, J. (1999) Supersister … speaking out. *Nursing Times* 95(21): 22.

Scott, P. (1987) Clinical leadership for staff nurses. *RNAO News* 43(4): 15.

Shepherd, E. (2000) What is the future of clinical leadership? *Nursing Times* 96(20): 40.

Sofarelli, D. Brown, D. (1998) The need for nursing leadership in uncertain times. *Journal of Nursing Management* 6: 201–207.

Stanley, D. (2006a) In command of care: clinical nurse leadership explored. *Journal of Research in Nursing* 11(1): 20–30.

Stanley, D. (2006b) In command of care: towards the theory of congruent leadership. *Journal of Research in Nursing* 11(2): 132–144.

Stanley, D. (2006c) Role conflict: leaders and managers. *Nursing Management* 13(5): 31–37.

Stanley, D. (2008) Congruent leadership: values in action. *Journal of Nursing Management* 16: 519–524.

Stogdill, R.M. (1974) *Handbook of Leadership*. New York: Free Press.

Strauss, A. Corbin, J. (1998) *Basics of Qualitative Research Techniques and Procedures for Developing Grounded Theory*. London: Sage.

Thyer, G. (2003) Dare to be different: transformational leadership may hold the key to reducing the nursing shortage. *Journal of Nursing Management* 11: 73–79.

Wedderburn-Tate, C. (1999) *Leadership in Nursing*. London: Churchill Livingstone.

Welford, C. (2002) Matching theory to practice. *Nursing Management* 9(4), 7–11.

Wilkinson, G. Miers, M. (eds) (1999) *Power and Nursing Practice*. London: Macmillan.

Wright, J. (1996) Unlock the leadership potential. *Nursing Management* 3(2): 8–10.

Wylie, K. (2008) Hospital crisis: 70 nurses needed. *The Press* (Christchurch, New Zealand), 29 February: A1.

8 Leadership for health globally: grasping the nettle

Veronica Bishop

Overview

Is leadership important to us – and if it is, why can't we grasp it? Drawing together the professional issues that pertain to non-medical health care providers, we reconsider their primary focus and purpose, particularly in the light of globalization. How may it impact on such a huge workforce? In this chapter we draw from previous chapters for a global audience – especially in countries where these professions are newly developing – highlighting where lessons can be learned and pitfalls avoided.

Introduction

Is leadership important to us – and if it is, why can't we grasp it? While the importance of health professionals participating in decision making at policy levels is stressed, so too is the difficulty in recruiting to key leadership roles both in the UK and in the wider community. It could be argued that any disenchantment that health care professionals may have with their leaders, or the perceived lack of them, reflects not so much on those in high places as on those who do not invest in themselves. It is time to draw together the professional issues that pertain to non-medical health care providers, to reconsider their primary focus and purpose. In all health care disciplines there are common dimensions, these being ethical, clinical and political, and all must – to be relevant and ethical – be underpinned by sound research.

Leaders must be aware of the bigger picture: What does globalization mean to nurses and allied health care professionals, and how may it impact on this huge workforce? More importantly, how can these health professions impact on global and national health service policies? In this chapter we reconsider where leadership is for nurses and allied health care professionals and, in the light of previous chapters, draw examples for a global audience – especially in those countries where these professions are newly developing – where lessons can be learned and pitfalls avoided.

Leadership functions

It might be useful at this stage to remind ourselves as to what a leader is, as opposed to a manager. A slick, quick definition that will keep us on the straight and narrow while we explore the entirety of what has gone before and look to the future is this:

> Leaders are focused on doing the right thing, whereas managers are focused on doing things right.
>
> (Detmar 1998: 101)

Alimo-Metcalfe and Alban-Metcalfe (2004) write that a leader should

- Provide continuity and momentum
- Be flexible in allowing changes of direction
- Ideally be a few steps ahead of their team, but not so far that the team cannot understand or follow.

In common with most critical writing of nurse leaders in the UK since the late 1970s is the perception that most were promoted for their allegiance with the status quo (Hamilton-Hurren 1997), and few recognized that power comes only from the empowerment of others (Farmer 1993: 36). The difficulties of this scenario, where individuals within a disenfranchised profession seek to empower other individuals, should not be underestimated. Bellman (2003) observes that empowerment has come to a minority of nurses, and cites examples that mostly derive from a shortfall of medical practitioners. This poses the question: Is it appropriate for nurses to pick up work previously carried out by other members of the team? And if it is, is it also appropriate for those tasks previously carried out by nurses to be taken up by less qualified staff? Such blurring of professional identities is a double-edged sword, and in 2002 I asked the question in an editorial 'Has the nursing profession mapped out a course for its own development, or is it being manipulated to tread the paths of others? And if this is so, do we mind?' (Bishop 2002: 240). Subsequent work gathered on leadership revealed that while leadership was high on the national agenda, much of the research ongoing was small scale and further fuelled the general recognition that more needed to be done, that there was a perceived lack of leaders. A national initiative implemented at this time was the 'Leading an Empowered Organization' programme (LEO). This was designed to create a critical mass of clinical leaders with the ability to make a real difference to patient care, and promoted a transformational style of leadership (Woolnough and Faugier 2002). Again, the main focus of the participants appeared to be that of management rather than leadership, but none the less was generally valued. Similar findings were made by Werrett and her colleagues (Werrett et al. 2002), leading Wilson-Barnett (2002) to conclude that perhaps the time had come to identify leadership outcomes, and this concept is taken forward effectively by Antrobus and her colleagues in Chapter 5.

Harnessing power

Ours is a constantly changing world, where the past is small guide to the future and traditional hierarchies are unlikely to apply in an effective organization. The pace and scale of change can sometimes seem disorientating, with constantly shifting expectations, and ever accelerating technical innovations. This means leaders have to rely more than ever on their intuition, beliefs and vision, to connect with their peers, and be open to critique. The many controversies in health care produce profound uncertainties and ambiguities, not least in the areas of equity and access, issues with profound ethical implications. As the convenor of six groups meeting to discuss health issues Marinker (1994: 3) was impressed by three salient features of policy making in health care:

- The profound uncertainties and ambiguities in medicine that masquerade as facts
- The pervasiveness of conflicting ideas and values
- The complexity of the group process by which we come to an agreement about what to do.

I suspect that over a decade on he would find the complexities even greater!

Sometimes this can seem too much to take on, particularly in an overstretched service. Collinson (2002: 403) describes this feeling of dispiritedness well:

Think about a meeting you have been in about the future of your unit, service or organisation. You are aware that people are playing games, that there is clearly a hidden agenda, that no decisions are being made, and that the word 'patient' hasn't yet been mentioned. You remember leaving the room dispirited and powerless, and going to see what crisis has occurred while you were away. You wonder what time you will get home tonight.

These are the times when it is crucial to hold on to the good feelings; to remember why you chose the profession that you are in, and to reflect on the buzz you have felt when you achieved quality interventions with patients and colleagues. It is also the time to plan in a positive way how you might change your own input to prevent such a mechanistic and wasteful exercise occurring again. This is not easy. In her excellent synopsis of the context for nurse-led change and development, Bellman (2003) notes that nurses are socially conditioned to accept taken–for–granted cultural norms – institutional rules and routines that enable them to participate willingly in their own domination. However, she supports the view that I shared elsewhere (Bishop and Scott 2001) – that while nurses may believe that they have little power within the organization, they wield considerable power when caring for patients. Harnessing that power in a positive and constructive manner that facilitates professional growth for improved patient outcomes is where true professional leadership should be focusing. Saks (in Chapter 3) rightly highlights the professional closure techniques employed by professionals on both sides of the Atlantic (and no doubt elsewhere), which while masquerading as being for the public good were more inclined to the benefit of the professionals involved. Saks also cites examples of very practical leadership that have very positive knock-on effects for the public good. The first was the action of the American Nurses' Association against cost-cutting by supporting hospitals that have a good record of nurse retention, by giving them a special designation through its newly established American Nurses Credentialing Center. Second, some nursing associations are lobbying for, among other things, legislation to ensure minimum registered nurse–patient ratios and for more nurses for patients who need intensive nursing. While this will no doubt be seen as self-serving by some, the benefit for patient care should be apparent. It is having the courage to grasp the power that automatically accompanies those working with vulnerable people and to use it constructively that is key to professional progress and public good. Keyzer (1992) expressed it well stating:

Nursing must now face the reality that past professional strategies have denied it the power base in clinical practice. It now requires to promote leaders who will remain in clinical practice and to have its voice heard in the clinical decision-making process.

(Keyzer 1992: 86)

From rhetoric to practice

We have discussed at some length the global implication for health care delivery, and are aware of the political, economic, demographic and social environment in which we ourselves work. These dynamics impact on us all as individuals to a greater or lesser degree, and effect our contribution to care. Health professionals across the world require leadership that is empowering, enabling them to meet these challenges effectively and in a manner that supports the wishes of patients. One can only agree with Kitson (2002) that this move from rhetoric to practice will require a philosophical leap from a subservient stance to one that embraces initiative. Kitson's view of leadership is about knowing how to make visions become reality. Courses on managing change have abounded for some years now, but little has really changed. Why is this? Certainly a climate of short-term policies, of diminishing growth set against increased demand makes for a nervous and uninspiring society. Creating an environment where risk is blame-free, where innovation is allowed to fail, and where intellect is rewarded and retained is a challenge that has focused the mind of leaders of industry, health care, academia and policy. An example of this was a conference entitled 'Future Summit 2004: Creating a Better World', organized by the Australian government. Here invited participants from a broad range of expertise considered the way forward for Australia and the wider global community to achieve collaborative goals. This summit called for a shared vision, clarity of purpose, and for commitment from every individual, reflecting the foundations for any progressive movement.

Leaders are everywhere in society, not just at the top of organizations and government. More to the point, one does not have to be a recognized leader to instigate change. Instead, one has to own an issue, decide to deal with it, then act upon it. As Jeffery (2004) put it:

> We cannot necessarily be the best at everything we do, but we can do our best. If we want to take advantage of the wealth of knowledge of our people and their ability to be creative, then we will need to make some 'big bets and have a go'. And we might not always win either.
>
> (Jeffery 2004: 12)

Individual health care workers may feel that this is an unrealistic philosophy that does not, nor should not, relate to patient services. I would argue that this is avoidance. Further development and striving for excellence is what being an accountable health care professional is about. This serves not only to improve the life of, and the contribution of, the individual, but also touches everyone around, feeding into the culture and spilling into a newer world. Individual actions do count, and taking ownership of an issue, dealing with it – this is leadership.

Whether we speak of individual leadership at a small, local level, or of leadership within or across a large organization, there are overlapping foci that need to be recognized. It is interesting to note that Antrobus and her colleagues describe (in Chapter 5) three overlapping leadership domains, whereas I would select a slight variation, placing 'academic' as opposed to 'strategic/executive', both sets of domains however are linked by the recognition of global relevance.

Leadership domains: Antrobus et al.	**Leadership domains: Bishop**
● Clinical leadership	● Clinical leadership
● Strategic/executive leadership	● Academic leadership
● Political leadership	● Professional/political leadership
	Global leadership

The difference between strategic as opposed to academic is likely to be a reflection of our individual careers, alternatively the use of 'executive' may reflect the merging of management with leadership. Drawing on the previous chapters we will now consider these individually and consider how to use existing frameworks to maximize your contribution as a follower or a leader. All of the domains must be based on ethical principles, which we will explore first.

Ethics and leadership

There are basic frameworks in existence to support or dictate ethical behaviour, both in our personal lives and professionally; indeed they are mainly bound in statute. However, there are huge areas where the letter of the law may be kept, but the spirit of it fails crushingly. For example, historically nursing developed from a position of servitude where subservience to doctors was the rule. In developing its own professional leadership system nursing has carried this culture of hierarchical dominance and oppression with it, resulting in many of its leaders going unchallenged and becoming insular. Asbridge (2001: 18), who was appointed as the chief executive of the newly formed UK Nursing and Midwifery Council in 2004, considered that nursing has 'developed a system of oppressing its own because the nursing hierarchy couldn't cope with anything that was outside command and control'. Interestingly he did not choose to note that employers of nurses at that time were most likely to give senior posts to men! Farmer (1993) noted similarly that nurse leaders, in their hunger for personal aggrandisement, often acted at the expense of the common good. This is not the behaviour of any ethical group.

The ethical dimension of taking on a leadership role within a profession must reflect the Code of Practice of that discipline. At a series of focus groups

(Bishop and Scott 2001) held with nurses in a large general hospital, several of the participants felt that nursing had 'lost its way', and others saw it as a quasi-profession in that it had little autonomy, less apparent power and a history that does not reflect the established components of a profession, such as law and medicine. It was mooted that nursing still suffered from its 'below stairs' origins and had not yet developed the right culture to reflect sufficient progress in both clinical and political terms. Perhaps we should stop comparing ourselves with other professions, and unapologetically claim our place at the policy table – where would any health service be without us? It is time to let go of interesting but outdated and irrelevant baggage and accept that qualified AHPs meet the criteria of a profession as stated by Tawney (1921):

> The difference between industry and as it exists today, a profession is ... unmistakable. The essence of the former is that its only criterion is the financial return which it offers to its shareholders. The essence of the latter is that though men enter it for their livelihood, the measure of its success is the service which they perform, not the gain which they amass.
> (Tawney 1921: 94)

Professional leadership

Professional leadership must have a complementary but different focus from business leadership. Clearly both foci are essential when resources are limited and demands ever growing. Good leadership is about handling the essential differences in a manner that facilitates quality care with good housekeeping. Allowing a 'them and us' situation to predominate is as unhelpful to the aims of any health service as unquestioning subservience, and is far from the ideals of a profession based on ethical concepts. Saks (Chapter 3) highlights the counterproductive effects of tribalism at all levels of health care in modern Britain and the United States. Remarking on the negative impact this must have on relationships in health care, he emphasizes the knock-on effect this has on professional leadership. Not only are patients put at risk from diverted energies and poor communications, but also the concept of a profession – a mode of work that provides a service for the public good – is severely singed, and the phoenix rising from the ashes is little more than a self-serving vanity.

Lack of clarity will damage any leadership strategy, and leadership can become fractured and uncertain. Berwick (2004) posits that clinicians ought to be playing a central role in the making of policies in the health care system that will allow better outcomes, greater use of ease, lower cost and greater social justice. Britain is home to many cultures, yet a review of the literature and the discourse around cultural diversity in the UK portrays it to be a problem to be solved, rather than an opportunity to be realized. There are historic connotations for this, and regrettably, modern anxieties that in many cases prevent some people from minority ethnic communities seeking or receiving the care that they need and are entitled to. While there are some excellent initiatives in health care set up in order to provide culturally sensitive services, we have a long way to go in order to achieve equity (Bishop 2008), and will have to acknowledge and resolve many challenges to our perceptions of health and illness and to our behaviour. Creating a truly participative society is really about making social and cultural change and this is, as noted by Freshwater (2004: 241), especially difficult when there are multiple groups that feel they have been treated unfairly or excluded from mainstream society.

Accepting that our responses to the threat of illness and to treatment regimes is potentially influenced by the taken-for-granted ideas of our culture, as well as the medical-scientific knowledge that we are able to draw on by our engagement with education, the media and the health care system, Freshwater (2004) urges that this knowledge is not acquired for its own sake, but used to shape *our* behaviour, and to provide a political, institutional and individual practice which is inclusive and transformatory. As Freshwater and her colleagues note in Chapter 6, the former dependence on rules, regulations and policies is already being replaced with a strong orientation to the ethical and moral codes of human rights, which in turn will be shaped by the nature of the work communities of health professionals will create and do. This complements the views of Berwick (1994), who considers that currently most reforms in health care are actually changes in the surroundings rather than in the care itself, and makes a clarion call for professional organizations to embrace involvement in policymaking. Hargrove (1998) also argued for a more creative leadership style, one that matches a new agenda, with collaborative approaches and an awareness of the need to create a just society in a sustainable environment. Timely in this newly developing culture are the recommendations of the NHS Darzi interim and final reports (DoH 2007, 2008). These are discussed more fully under clinical leadership, and offer would-be clinical leaders new opportunities. While it is indisputable that any government has a responsibility to facilitate the creation of an environment and culture that supports the aspirations of clinicians and managers to provide first-class health care for patients, many of the problems within the NHS may not be laid at the door of the government health department, though they are certainly not guilt free! It can cogently be argued that the professions themselves get the government health department that they deserve.

Clinical leadership

Although the term clinical leadership seems to have originated in nursing, it is now being applied more widely across the whole range of clinicians, from doctors and nurses to all the professions allied to medicine. Recent activities in England have sought to explore how best to encourage clinicians and practitioners to take on leadership roles in the health sector. Arguably, this has been precipitated by the poor performance of some services in looking after the safety and well-being of patients while pursuing government performance targets. The unwanted increase in hospital-acquired infections and poor standards of cleanliness are prime examples of this blurred focus. *It is clear that clinical leadership will become a new mantra quite quickly*. How to achieve change is another question. The expert clinician needs help to be a leader.

Conclusions drawn from a conference (DoH 1993, 1994) attended by senior UK nurses in 1993 on taking the profession into the next century, identified six constants, which in my view apply to all health care professionals. These draw upon a tradition of caring, based around both skills and values and include:

- A co-ordinating function
- A teaching function, for carers, patients and professionals
- Developing and maintaining programmes of care
- Technical expertise, exercised personally and through others
- Concern for the ill, but also for those who are currently well
- A special responsibility for the frail and vulnerable.

These constants fit well with the ideology of a profession, promoting the interests of patients or clients and of the wider public. While individuals strive to meet these professional criteria, the importance of local leadership in supporting practitioners cannot be underestimated. The stress on all health care workers from the impact of an increasingly demanding and very disparate population are compounded by fragmented services and funding arrangements. Local leaders can, if properly focused and clear in their intent, provide that oft-needed clarity, encouragement or information. A 'have a go' mentality has to go hand in glove with a supportive blame-free organization and clinical supervision can be invaluable here in providing a series of clinically focused relationships that support knowledgeable practitioners (Bishop 2007a). Local leaders can be staff nurses or ward sisters as well as matrons or specialist nurses – being a champion of good care is not only the prerogative of status. A good example of this comes from the sporting world. Ian Botham played a blistering game of cricket in Australia, significantly contributing to the winning of the Ashes for England; he was a class player and no doubt inspirational within the team – but he was not the captain.

Leadership in the health sector in the UK has now reached a new stage in its development. It is fairly safe to say that the interests of potential health service managers now sit on a well-founded system which is among one of the best in the world. The NHS Institute for Innovation and Improvement (www.institute.nhs.uk) has recently reported on the significantly high quality of its health management graduate entry scheme such that it scores very highly against all other sectors that might bear comparison. This suggests that young graduates entering the health sector are among the highest calibre to be found. Yet the sector continues to suffer from poor leadership and underperformance in some areas, with government targets and the term 'effectiveness' used slavishly and often in isolation from the lived experience. Pearson (1998: 25) considers that 'excellent nursing' is a far broader concept than 'effective nursing', stating that the desired outcomes in terms of health status can be achieved in spite of the nursing that we provide – even if the care dehumanizes patients or devalues their experience. So while it is not possible to have excellent care without effectiveness, it is possible to be effective without being excellent.

The news on management and leadership is mixed but can nonetheless hold its head fairly high in broader public sector provision. A more vigorous debate is emerging on clinical leadership which looks to another part of the workforce to lead, innovate and manage. The recent activities of the Darzi second stage review in England (DoH 2008) have sought to explore how best to encourage clinicians and practitioners to take on leadership roles in the health sector. Interestingly Lord Darzi, a surgeon, is advocating that the locus of control moves from the centre (government) to local communities, in particular towards clinicians and patients themselves – stating that the centre should 'support local change not instruct it'. He also recommends moving the focus from the quantitative business of targets to the qualitative business of a 'relentless' focus on improving the quality of care and the quality of the patient experience of care. Acknowledging the many negative perceptions of the public, the disillusionment of staff, and lack of clout felt by patients, the report is structured into five areas for improvement: equity, personalization, outcomes, safety and local accountability, and will be tackled by stakeholders within eight specific types of care. Lovegrove (in Chapter 4) cites examples of clinical leadership that are innovative and allow for the full potential of the professionals involved to be tapped. If AHPs grasp the nettle and network with appropriate stakeholders a real opportunity for change may be presented here.

Expert clinicians need help to become leaders, and the opportunity to consider how best they can function in their local environment as a 'mover and shaker'. While many nurse authors support the view of Hargrove (1998) in the move from a hierarchical leadership style to one of consensus, this leadership style is not without its 'elephant traps'. A creative, collaborative model of leadership can work only if someone, somewhere, has sought a consensus that can be shaped into a strategy. This is where value judgements of differing professions and managerial priorities come into play, and where the politically unprepared player will let themselves down.

Similarly, as has been noted in previous chapters, there is currently a strong move to support the notion of transformational leadership as the preferred style to effect change in these fast-moving times, as it is seen to encourage innovation and change. However, there are ethical considerations when embracing change. This is where a good research and development underpinning is essential; evidence is hard currency. Clinical leadership will be ill-served if it is not in collaboration with academic leadership and political strength.

Academic leadership

Academia in the AHPs has been a piecemeal business, with nursing having the longest history and thus more time to organize its educational requirements, an exercise that is still ongoing and, given the dynamics of society is likely to remain so. McKenna and Galvin (2004) concur with Lanara (1994) in considering that members of any profession are best able to appreciate the essence of their discipline when their educational programme includes not only studying but also generating, challenging and testing the knowledge in their field, and they make a strong case for the scholarly practitioner with doctoral qualifications. They note that in countries where nurses have been delayed in gaining admission to doctoral programmes the development of nursing knowledge has also been delayed. Sherwood and Freshwater (2005: 58) are concerned with such matters, and in drawing specific attention to nurse leadership argue that:

> Doctoral education is charged with preparing leaders who can think out of the box and stimulate creative problem solving in others invigorating nurses to claim a voice in crafting a vision of health care delivery that recognizes the essentialness of nursing.

This is not the moment to argue for or against a degree-only profession, but what is indisputable is that any professional group must have the resource of sound research to support its practice. Freshwater and Graham examine this in more detail in Chapter 6 and Butterworth sets out new developments (Butterworth 2009) that have good potential for academic developments if clear leadership prevails.

Focusing on a truly expansive approach to nursing knowledge, Freshwater and Picard (2004: 45) observe that nursing care is a global concern and the movement of people across national boundaries makes it important that the understanding of health and nursing care problems is examined and shared internationally. This requires a cadre of academics to undertake both the teaching and research aspects of the profession. However, despite the movement of schools of nursing in the UK from hospitals to institutions of higher education in the 1990s, and the growth of around 80 schools of nursing within universities, employers of educators and researchers in health and social care faced a critical shortfall of staff. This had been brought about by disparities in pay and reward and rigid or poorly articulated career opportunities, and while the problem was evident in most areas of social and health care, it was most severe in nursing. Chaired by Butterworth, a cross-government departments committee was set up to identify the academic workforce problems and to make recommendations for an academic human resource plan to support learning and research in health and social care (StLAR) which is described fully by Butterworth et al. (2005). One of the most important problems within the academic environment is that teaching is often perceived as being of lesser importance than research, thus undermining the adage that research should inform teaching and teaching, in turn, informs practice (McKenna 2005). Many initiatives seeking to bridge the much bewailed practice–theory gap have been tried out, such as lecturer–practitioner roles. Sometimes they have worked well, but as is often the case, the success or failure depends greatly on the individual's commitment and the support of the employing agencies.

Despite this, leadership in academic nursing has quite a healthy global profile, with collaborative work crossing often unlikely boundaries. How great the impact of academia is on practice across the world is far more difficult to ascertain. Journals flourish, dissemination is rewarded by research funding and professional recognition, but the recipe for getting research into practice is an elusive one. Johnson (2004) strongly argues that nursing research had lost its way, and had forgotten how to discover the truth about the realities of nursing and other forms of patient care. While I have made a case for clinical governance being an asset to nursing (Bishop 2007b), Johnson (2004) considers that the profession has become hamstrung by it and lost perspective on the actual harms and benefits involved in nursing research. We have approached clinical governance from different perspectives, and I value his well-presented views on its relevance to research. Such discussions should be easily available to health care staff generally and to academic staff in particular. As modern technology has changed dramatically how libraries function, to the benefit of users, and as the future of nursing depends on research-based practices local leaders should ensure that up-to-date data are available. As I have noted previously (Bishop 1994):

The harnessing of the potential within the nursing profession to make a major impact on the quality of care is indeed a challenge. It is a challenge that has triggered many initiatives both large and small, research based and practice driven. Nursing research is not the prerogative of an elite few; it belongs to the profession and must be bedded into practice.

(Bishop 1994: 194)

Because of the complexity of nursing work we need to consider new approaches to evaluating our care. Normand (2004) notes that while a plethora of studies has been carried out in an attempt to empower staff to use research findings, others argue that there is a need for the gap between research and practice to be strategically addressed rather than through focus on the individual practitioner. It is to be hoped that the recently published *State of the Art Metrics for Nursing* (Griffiths et al. 2008) heralds a robust infrastructure that will place patient-centred (rather than disease-centred) research firmly in the clinical arena, thus addressing the need to integrate nursing into clinical governance.

Political leadership

At a nurses' conference in 2007 former UK health minister and Conservative peer Baroness Cumberlege told participants that it was high time nurses became more politically aware, adding that to do so, they need to understand the psychological differences between their profession and politicians. She stated:

"Nurses are scientific. When they want to get to the core of a problem they always try to drill down. Yet politics are about the big picture. Nurses are agriculturalists in that they grow and nurture things but politicians are hunters – they're always after the big game. It's these kinds of differences nurses need to start to understand."

(Cumberlege 2007)

I recall discussions with the Baroness at a briefing meeting when she was still a serving minister and I was a government nursing officer; we were considering the best way for her to approach an interview the following day, and eventually, after we had viewed the uppermost issue of the day from every angle she said 'Oh, nursing is so big!' How right she was – there is hardly any aspect of life that it does not overlap or impinge on, so considering the big picture is a mammoth task! And again, she is right, we need leaders who have clarity and energy, and can cut through the detail and focus on the professional entity. A frequent observation made about nursing advocacy at the policy level is its absence – or at least its invisibility (Spenceley et al. 2006), despite a persistent belief that nurses will participate in advocacy at the societal level in matters of health.

One of the problems with the nursing profession is that while there are nearly 11 million nurses in the world, and they certainly make up the largest workforce in the NHS in the UK, if not globally, it is mainly female dominated. There is no doubt in my mind that in a mainly male-dominated world women do have to work twice as hard as their male counterparts, and be twice as convincing. This is illustrated time and again on televised political news programmes, where male and female interviewers frequently present a far more aggressive or dismissive approach to female interviewees, no matter what their status. Here is not the place for a discourse on feminism, but there must be sympathy for the view put forward by Davies (2004) that the central predicament of nursing as a woman's occupation in a man's world remains unresolved. This view is strongly upheld by Salvage and Smith (2000), who consider that the marginalization not only of nursing but also of the values it traditionally represents lies in part from doctors' – a male-dominated profession – ignorance about it. However, this editorial goes on to remark that the rules of the (power) game are changing, with today's nurses being more assertive and well educated, while the doctors are less certain of their ground. I suspect that the old 'doctor versus nurse' notion is almost dead and that far more relevant nowadays are the pressures brought to bear on all health care professionals of consumerism, general management and political short-termism.

Political awareness, and turning that into useful action, is unlikely to occur without guidance; it is a road littered with pitfalls that can delete future negotiations before they commence. When I worked in the Department of Health, in collaboration with the then Women's Unit, we promoted the concept of 'shadowing', where aspiring leaders shadowed senior members of either their employing authority or their selected government agency. While very limiting in that too many people might want to shadow the very small number of senior staff, it was a move in the right direction. Far more manageable is the approach taken by Antrobus and her colleagues, as described in Chapter 5. Having identified four approaches to the politics of care – awareness, astuteness, action and finally political leadership – Antrobus and her colleagues illustrate with excellent case studies how to move from the beginning towards the climax of this journey.

Global impacts and organizational tensions

In commenting on the global changes of the then forthcoming millennium, Bottery (1998) describes how smaller communities and cultures have attempted to assert their identities by breaking away from historic larger states. Examples of this range from the break up of the old Soviet Union to the United Kingdom, where devolution is high on the agenda and decentralization a policy statement. Despite this, Bottery (1998) saw this millennium as the age of the larger grouping, and considers that these changes have come hard for many. He argues that health care professionals (and others) must understand the implications of globalization if they do not wish to be reduced to mere 'functionaries' in a larger institutional and managerial scheme in which notions of public good are increasingly traded for institutional success. This can be hard for people who elected to work for a health service that had been designed for the public good rather than for the criteria of the marketplace, those of economy and efficiency. The term globalization is banded about with little thought as to how it differs from 'internationalization', so let us define our terms. *International* implies the sovereignty of individual nations, and agreements between various groups. *Global* opens the door to new forms of policy in which decisions are made and supported by global laws that transcend pooled national interests.

If we are to understand where our future lies (not only in health care but also in society as a whole) we need to appreciate the new range of challenges that arise from a move from nationally focused approaches of care to global ones. The changing nature of disease worldwide – with the resurgence of previously controlled diseases such as tuberculosis, and pandemics of newer viruses such as bird influenza and SARS – requires half-forgotten skills to be revived, and new ones to be learned. The United Nations (2008) Millennium Development Goals make international calls for strengthening health systems, for the renewed focus on primary health and community-based care, and for focus on trends in obesity and chronic, non-communicable diseases. The range of global challenges, from eradicating extreme poverty and hunger to halting the spread of HIV/AIDS and providing universal primary education, all by the target date of 2015, form a blueprint for all the world's countries and leading development institutions. However, blueprints, to be successful, require leadership and global health requires leadership that respects evidence, that actively promotes learning within disciplines and engineers effective collaboration. Garrett (2007) notes that in 1997 the biggest problem in global health was lack of available resources to combat the multiple scourges ravaging the world's poor and sick. Today the recent unprecedented rise in public and private charitable donations has resulted in more money being directed towards pressing heath challenges than ever before. However, Garrett and other writers (e.g. Buchan 2002, 2004) have highlighted the fact that there is a worldwide shortage of health care workers, coupled with a disproportionate concentration of health workers in developed nations and urban areas. So despite the generous funding available, the lack of an educated workforce stands in the way of achieving such key public health priorities as reducing child and maternal mortality, increasing vaccine coverage, and battling epidemics such as HIV/AIDS. This situation is exacerbated by the ageing populations of the developed countries who need ever more medical attention and entice away local health talent from developing countries. While the ethics of this have been bandied about for some time (e.g. Aiken et al. 2004; Xu and Zhang 2005), a study published in 2007 estimated that if current trends continue, by 2020 the United States could face a shortage of up to 800,000 nurses and 200,000 doctors (Kuehn 2007). It is the view of that author that unless the United States and other wealthy nations radically increase salaries and domestic training programmes for physicians and nurses, it is likely that within 15 years the majority of workers staffing their hospitals will have been born and trained in poor and middle-income countries. As such workers flood to the West, the developing world will grow even more desperate.

There is a view that the visionary leadership needed at a global level to tackle such problems is sadly lacking (Garrett 2007). Awareness of the problems associated with migrating staff has caused the International Council of Nurses (ICN 2002), and more recently Sigma Theta Tau International (2005), a US-based honour society, to highlight the issue in their position statements. In these they confirm the right of nurses to migrate, and note the potential beneficial outcomes of multicultural practice and learning opportunities supported by migration, but emphasize that the potential adverse effect on quality of health care in donor countries has not been addressed adequately. In the UK a paradox currently exists where many home-educated newly qualified AHPs and nurses are unable to find work within their discipline and are forced to leave the health services while non-UK staff are actively sought. The Crisp Report (2007) makes recommendations which could, if implemented, offer opportunities for short-term employment abroad and facilitate hands-on exchange of skills and learning. His view of global partnerships is encouraging and puts parochialism with the dinosaurs:

> We also increasingly share in the threats and challenges of global health – and global disease – and with our increasingly diverse population need to understand the diseases, genetic predispositions and cultures of, for example, Sub-Saharan Africa and South Asia if we are to look after our own population well. There are things we can learn from each other in all of these areas. There are partnerships we can create and strengthen between countries and between communities and individuals. Over time we can perhaps start to emphasise more the similarities between us, rather than the differences – and even stop using the words 'developing' and 'developed'.
>
> (Crisp 2007: 25)

While clearly no one country has all the answers to the worldwide health care dilemmas we face today, with such extremes as obesity to lack of access to clean drinking water, the need to work together and to pool skills has never been more important. In a numbers game – where there is potential for power – health care professionals have a head start, yet lack the status. Strong collaborative leadership could build a united and cohesive group that would be effective in influencing policy.

The World Health Organization repeatedly advocates the strengthening of nursing and midwifery leadership, following its resolution in 1992 (WHO 1992), and this clarion call has been sounded across its large membership by the International Council of Nurses, the oldest and largest association of health professionals in the world. In the WHO publication *A Resource for Better Health*, Ralph et al. (1997) cite the 1993 Commonwealth Secretariat draft document that stated:

> Nurse and midwives must play a full part in key policy and planning decisions. The knowledge which comes from their practice places them in a privileged position to bring decision making at ministerial and government level, and to boards of management of health services in the public and private sectors, that perspective of service delivery without which decisions are often flawed.
>
> (Commonwealth Secretariat 1993, quoted in Ralph et al. 1997: 172)

Despite this apparent support from potentially powerful allies, leadership in the non-medical health professions has been at best patchy and, at worse, illusory.

Conclusion

From Chapter 1, where the different (and differing) concepts of leadership are unpicked, we moved on in Chapter 2, to the often ignored but highly significant difference between leadership and management. I share the view of Stanley that all AHPs (and many others) have been held back from maximizing their leadership roles by a lack of understanding of these two concepts. It is a difficult area and one that many authors baulk at and skim over – to the reader's loss. I suspect that one of the many reasons for medicine's persistent domination of health care policy is the lack of professional clarity needed here. Saks (in Chapter 3) takes us into the domains of turf wars between professions, won in the main on both sides of the Atlantic by our medical colleagues, and importantly highlights the ethical dimensions of professional self-interest and advancement for the public good.

This picks up one of the issues raised by Antrobus et al. in Chapter 5, where they describe four stages of leadership derived from Cohen et al. (1996) and go further in proposing a fifth stage – global leadership. The impact of fast developing countries on older health care systems is already shaking traditional systems, for example with patients travelling from the UK to India for open heart surgery. The growth of nursing in China cannot but impact on current systems. Health care practice is influenced by socio-economic-political contexts, and so is nursing practice. Although Hong Kong has returned to China, under the 'one country two system policy' Hong Kong has retained its own system of nursing development. It is difficult to merge the two nursing systems because of the different health care needs in both societies. The development of nursing in mainland China is much government driven, where there are about 1.5 million nurses. There is no doubt that they could exert an important influence in the health care system if they were united. Hong Kong nurses have better ability to read and write in English, which facilitates the sharing and networking with other parts of the world. This collaboration is important for the future development of nursing in the East, and how they will interact with the rest of the world. The focus in Singapore on recruitment and improved status of AHPs described in Chapter 4 offers ideas for other countries to improve recruitment and retention.

Valuing tacit knowledge

Difficulties arise in nursing and with its paramedical colleagues in that much of its knowledge is tacit. While major funding for research is mostly available for biomedical research – despite most health care being delivered in teams of many disciplines – so defining outcomes and achieving further professional status is only achieved by a few researchers. Freshwater (2004) urges universities not only to ensure that research is undertaken that is driven by community priorities and excellence, but also to take more risks. She adds that permission to fail may encourage researchers to push frontiers and challenge old ways of working. Freshwater highlights the trickle-down effect of highly innovative individuals in their midst: keeping such people attracts other like-minded individuals and creates a collegiate community. Academia has to remember, too, that it is not self-serving, but must relate meaningfully to the services of its discipline. Likewise, services providers must think beyond finance. The argument for the management mantra of economy, efficiency and effectiveness has to be balanced in a public service by a realistic vision from professionals who have hands-on, practical understanding of what that service is about. While health care cannot exist in isolation from resource allocation, legislation and management, neither can it effectively function if its workforce have, from force of habit, ceased to be people who think of any greater good.

Final thoughts

The reason that there are so many leadership books is because it is a highly complex subject, and as such is prone to exciting new ideas and semantics. I hope that within the text of this book, the contributors have managed to stimulate and substantiate a sound basis for your individual progress on the leadership journey. I hope also that you have been irritated – it will show that previously held concepts have been shaken, if not stirred!

Pearson (1998: 27) commented on nurses' tendency to polarize, which prevents us from moving forward. It is, as he suggested in 1988, time to sit down and be more open with each other and see if we can move forward and mature into a group that values knowledge in all its various guises. Walter Lippmann (1945) wrote that the sign of a good leader was that their ideas carried on after they had gone. I would rather call that the role of a philosopher. I see leaders as being the people who provide the constant energy to bring the philosophy alive, to make it pertinent to today and tomorrow, and maybe, to change it.

Key points

- Leaders in health care must invest in themselves, as well as using established organizational opportunities.
- Leaders must take personal ownership of strategies and actions.
- Health professionals' power must be based on research-based clinical excellence.
- A blame-free culture would encourage risk taking based on sound knowledge.
- A leader makes known a shared vision, owns it and knows how to achieve it.

References

Aiken, L.H., Buchan, J., Sochalski, J., Nichols, B. and Powell, M. (2004) Trends in international nurse migration: the world's wealthy countries must be aware of how the 'pull' of nurses from developing countries affects global health. *Health Affairs* 23(3): 69–77.

Alimo-Metcalfe, B. and Alban-Metcalfe, J. (2004) Leadership: time for a new direction? Leadership 1(1): 51–71.

Asbridge, J. (2001) Share deal. *Nursing Standard* 15(17): 17–18.

Bellman, L. (2003) *Nurse-led Change and Development in Clinical Practice*. London: Whurr.

Berwick, D.M. (1994) Eleven worthy aims for clinical leadership of health system reform. *Journal of the American Medical Association* 272(10): 797–802.

Berwick, D. (2004) *NHS Live Master Class*: www.doh.gov.uk.

Bishop, V. (1994) Prevention and primary health care delivery challenges. In J.J. Fitzpatrick, J.S. Stevenson and N.S. Polis (eds) *Nursing Research and its Utilisation*. New York: Springer.

Bishop, V. (2002) Editorial. *Journal of Research in Nursing* 7(4): 240.

Bishop, V. (2007a) Clinical supervision: What is it? Why do we need it? In V. Bishop (ed.) *Clinical Supervision in Practice: Some Questions, Answers and Guidelines for Professionals in Health and Social Care*, 2nd edn. Basingstoke: Palgrave Macmillan.

Bishop, V. (2007b) Clinical supervision: functions and goals. In V. Bishop (ed.) *Clinical Supervision in Practice; Some Questions, Answers and Guidelines for Professionals in Health and Social Care*, 2nd edn. Basingstoke: Palgrave Macmillan.

Bishop, V. (2008) Editorial. *Journal of Research in Nursing* 13: 3–5.

Bishop, V. and Scott, I. (2001) Introduction. In V. Bishop and I. Scott (eds) *Challenges in Clinical Practice: Professional Developments in Nursing*. Basingstoke: Palgrave Macmillan.

Bottery, M. (1998) *Professionals and Policy: Management Strategy in a Competitive World*. London: Cassell.

Buchan, J. (2002) Editorial. Global nursing shortages. *British Medical Journal* 324: 751–752.

Buchan, J. (2004) Challenges of recruiting and retaining nurses: some thoughts for policy makers. *Journal of Research in Nursing* 8(4): 291–292.

Butterworth T. (2009) Board Editorial *Journal of Research in Nursing* 14: 2

Butterworth, A., Jackson, C., Brown, E., Hessey, E., Fergusson, J. and Orme, M. (2005) Clinical academic careers for educators and researchers in nursing. *Journal of Research in Nursing* 10(1): 85–98.

Cohen, S., Mason, D., Kovner, C., Leavitt, J., Pulcinin, J. and Sochalski, J. (1996) Stages of nursing's political development: where we've been and where we ought to go. *Nursing Outlook* 44: 259–266.

Collinson, G. (2002) The primacy of purpose and the leadership of nursing. *Nursing Times Research* 7(6): 403–411.

Commonwealth Secretariat (1993) *Challenges and Opportunities: Draft Framework for Action*. London: Commonwealth Secretariat.

Crisp, N. (2007) *Global Health Partnerships: The UK Contribution to Health in Developing Countries* (Crisp Report). London: Central Office of Information: www.dfid.gov.uk/pubs/files/ghp.pdf.

Cumberlege, J. (2007) Speech quoted in 'Has nursing leadership lost its way?' *Healthcare Republic* 5 February.

Davies, C. (2004) Political leadership and the politics of nursing. *Journal of Nursing Management* 12: 235–241.

Department of Health (DoH) (1993) *The Heathrow Debate*. London: DoH.

Department of Health (1994) *Heathrow Debate: The Challenges for Nursing and Midwifery in the 21st. Century*. London: DoH.

Department of Health (2007) *Our NHS, Our Future: Interim Report, England* (Darzi Report). London: DoH.

Department of Health (2008) *High Quality Care for All* (Darzi Report). London: DoH.

Detmar, S. (1998) Clinical leadership in nursing: the RN as integrator. In J. Rocchiccioli and M.S. Tilbury (eds) *Clinical Leadership in Nursing*. Philadelphia, PA: Saunders.

Farmer, B. (1993) The use and abuse of power in nursing. *Nursing Standard* 7(23): 33–36.

Freshwater, D. (2004) A tool for clinical leadership? *Reflections on Nursing Leadership* 30(2): 20–26.

Freshwater, D. and Picard, C. (2004) International perspectives: collaborative conversations. In D. Freshwater and V. Bishop (eds) *Nursing Research in Context: Appreciation, Application and Professional Development*. Basingstoke: Palgrave Macmillan.

Garrett, L. (2007) The challenge of global health. *Foreign Affairs* January–February. New York: Council on Foreign Relations.

Griffiths, P., Jones, S., Maben, J. and Murrels, T. (2008) *State of the Art Metrics for Nursing: A Rapid Appraisal*. London: King's College London.

Hamilton-Hurren, A. (1997) Empowerment. *Nursing in Critical Care* 2(3): 109–110.

Hargrove, R. (1998) *Mastering the Art of Creative Collaboration*. New York: McGraw-Hill.

International Council of Nurses (2002) *Position Statement on Nurse Migration*: www.icn.ch.

Jeffery, M. (2004) *Report of the First Annual Future Summit*, Sydney, 6–8 May: www.futuresummit.org.

Johnson, M. (2004) Real-world ethics and nursing research. *Journal of Research in Nursing* 9(4): 251–261.

Keyzer, D. (1992) Nursing policy: the supply and demand for nurses. In J. Robinson, A. Gray and R. Elkan (eds) *Policy Issues in Nursing*. Buckingham: Open University Press.

Kitson, A. (2002) Nursing leadership: bringing caring back to the future. *Policy, Politics & Nursing Practice* 3(2): 108–117.

Kuehn, B.M. (2007) Global shortage of health workers, brain drain stress developing countries. *Journal of American Medical Association* 298: 1853–1855.

Lanara, V.A. (1994) The contribution of nursing research to the development of the discipline of nursing in Europe. *Proceedings from the Seventh Biennial Conference*, Oslo, Workgroup of European Researchers.

Lippmann, W. (1945) *New York Herald Tribune* 14 April.

McKenna, H. (2005) Commentary. Research outputs, environment and esteem. *Journal of Research in Nursing* 10(6): 597–601.

McKenna, H. and Galvin, K. (2004) Doctoral processes. In D. Freshwater and V. Bishop (eds) *Nursing Research in Context; Appreciation, Application and Professional Development*. Basingstoke: Palgrave Macmillan.

Marinker, M. (1994) *Controversies in Health Care Policies: Challenges to Practice*. London: BMJ Publishing Group.

Normand, C. (2004) Commentary. Encouraging and not discouraging nursing research. *Journal of Research in Nursing* 9(6): 462–463.

Pearson, A. (1998) Excellence in care: future dimensions for effective nursing. *Journal of Research in Nursing* 3(1): 25–27.

Ralph, C., Salvage, J. and Ashton, R. (1997) The role of nurses and midwives in government. In J. Salvage and S. Heijnen (eds) *Nursing in Europe: A Resource for Better Health*. Copenhagen: World Health Organization.

Salvage, J. and Smith, R. (2000) Editorials. Doctors and nurses: doing it differently. *British Medical Journal* 320: 1019–1020.

Sherwood, G. and Freshwater, D. (2005) Doctoral education for transformational leadership in a global context. In S. Ketefian and H. McKenna (eds) *Doctoral Education in Nursing: International Perspectives*. London: Routledge.

Sigma Theta Tau International (2005) *Position Statement*: www.nursingsociety.org.

Spenceley, S., Reutter, L. and Allen, M. (2006) The road less traveled: nursing advocacy at the policy level. *Policy, Politics, and Nursing Practice* 7(3): 180–194.

Tawney, R.H. (1921) *The Acquisitive Society*. New York: Harcourt Brace.

United Nations (2008) UN Millennium Development Goals: www.un.org/millenniumgoals/.

Werrett, J.A., Griffiths, M. and Clifford, C. (2002) An Evaluation of the West Midlands Leading an Empowered Organisation Programme. Birmingham: School of Health Sciences, University of Birmingham.

Wilson-Barnett, J. (2002) Commentary. *Journal of Research in Nursing* 7(6): 471–472.

Woolnough, H. and Faugier, J. (2002) An evaluative study assessing the impact of the leading an empowered organisation programme. *Journal of Research in Nursing* 7(6): 421–427.

World Health Organization (1992) *Strengthening Nurses and Midwives in Support of Strategies of Health for All*. World Health Assembly Resolution WHA 45.5. Geneva: WHO.

Xu, Y. and Zhang, J. (2005) One size doesn't fit all: ethics of international nurse recruitment from the conceptual framework of stakeholder interests. *Nursing Ethics* 12(6): 571–581.

Index

EFFECTIVE PRACTICE IN HEALTH, SOCIAL CARE AND CRIMINAL JUSTICE 2E

A Partnership Approach

Ros Carnwell and Julian Buchanan (eds)

'Contemporary health and social care requires practitioners to develop effective partnerships with patients and clients and with the wider service workforce. This text is designed to promote the development of such partnerships and demonstrates the ways in which partnership can work effectively in practice ... This text is clearly written with all the health and social care professions in mind and will prove to be an invaluable resource for students and trained staff alike.'

Margaret Chambers, Lecturer in Children's Nursing, University of Plymouth, UK

Comprehensive yet concise, this text addresses many of the main social and health issues facing society today, and incorporates a practical focus to demonstrate partnership working. The new edition of this popular book has been updated to include new chapters on the partnership approach in criminal justice and provides a practical and theoretical insight into some of the issues when working in collaborative partnership with other agencies.

The text examines the partnership approach to delivering services in relation to:

- Child protection
- Mental health
- Gypsy travellers
- Domestic violence
- Drug misuse
- Homelessness
- Old and young people
- HIV and AIDS

The first section of the book examines the nature of partnership in relation to concepts, politics, diversity, ethics and information technology. The second edition incorporates knowledge from a range of carefully selected contributors, using their expertise with particular user groups to illustrate where collaboration is crucial for effective practice. The final section reflects upon what has been learnt about partnership work and includes reflections from a service user and a chapter on evaluation.

Effective Practice in Health, Social Care and Criminal Justice is an essential text for students, practitioners and managers from a variety of human service agencies, and is a must-read for anyone working in a multi-agency partnership.

Contents: *Notes on the contributors – Foreword by Walid El Ansari – Preface – Part I: The context of partnerships – The concepts of partnership and collaboration – The impact of the digital age on partnership and collaboration – Promoting inclusive partnership working – Ethical issues of working in partnership – Part II: Partnerships in practice – Inter-professional communication in child protection – Working in partnership to support people with mental health difficulties – Working across the interface of formal and informal care of older people – Understanding and misunderstanding problem drug use: Working together – Addressing homelessness through effective partnership working – Problem drug use and safeguarding children: Partnership and practice issues – Tackling behavioural problems in the classroom using a student assistance programme – Not behind closed doors: Working in partnership against domestic violence – Working with Gypsy Travellers: A partnership approach – Effective partnerships to assist mentally disordered offenders – Partnership approaches to working with people with HIV – Part III: Learning from partnerships – On the receiving end: Reflections from a service user – Evaluating partnerships – Learning from partnerships: Themes and issues – Developing best practice in partnership – References – Index.*

2008 312pp

978-0-335-22911-6 (Paperback)

THE HANDBOOK FOR ADVANCED PRIMARY CARE NURSES

Rebecca Neno and Debby Price (eds)

'*I believe that* The Handbook for Advanced Primary Care Nurses *should be extensively read and that it will prove to be an essential resource for nurses striving to improve public health and patient care in the communities of today and tomorrow. It may, with political will and a skilled and determined workforce help Florence Nightingale's vision come true.*'

Lynn Young, Primary Health Care Adviser, Royal College of Nursing, UK

This important new handbook for Primary Care Nurses is designed to assist senior nurses in developing the understanding and skills required to be effective at both strategic and operational levels. As well as exploring the context of advanced primary care practice, the book provides the tools needed for enhancing care delivery within both primary care and community settings.

The Handbook for Advanced Primary Care Nurses is an accessible guide to working strategically in primary care. It offers practical support across a range of core areas, including:

- Case finding and case management
- Mentorship
- Leadership and management
- Needs assessment
- Interprofessional working
- Prescribing

Neno and Price encourage readers to think analytically about their practice and include activities and reflection points throughout the book to help with this.

This book is the ideal companion both for nurse practitioners undertaking courses at advanced practice level and for professionals working at all levels in primary care.

Contents: Foreword – Contributors – Introduction – Part 1: Context – Emergence of the advanced primary care nurse – Part 2: Enhancing care delivery – Legal and ethical issues in advanced practice – Case finding – Case management – First contact and complex needs assessment – Non-medical prescribing – Part 3: Enhancing strategic skills – Developing whole systems thinking – Transformational leadership – Developing and sustaining the advanced practitioner role – Developing and sustaining professional partnerships – From involvement to partnerships and beyond Part 4: Developing skills for the future – Commissioning in health and social care – Social enterprise and business skills – Influencing and getting your message across – Part 5: Future directions – The future for advanced primary care nurses – Index.

2008 224pp

978-0-335-22353-4 (Paperback) 978-0-335-22354-1 (Hardback)